Health Service Finance
An Introduction

Health Service Finance
An Introduction

TOM JONES, BA. FCCA. IPFA. DMS
Treasurer for Herefordshire Health Authority

MALCOLM PROWLE, BSc. MA. FCCA. IPFA
Senior Management Consultant with Coopers and Lybrand Associates

with a Foreword by the Rt. Hon. Lord Ennals
Former Secretary of State for Social Services (1976-79)

Published by
The Certified Accountants Educational Trust
29 Lincoln's Inn Fields, London WC2A 3EE

This book has been prepared on behalf of the Certified Accountants Educational Trust
by Tom Jones and Malcolm Prowle.
The views expressed are those of the authors and not necessarily those of the Trust.

Jones, Tom
Health Service Finance - 2nd Ed.
i. Medical Care - England - Finance
I. Title II. Prowle, Malcolm
388.4,33621,0942   RA410.55.G7
ISBN 0-9000-94-540

Printed by: Walters Design and Print Services Limited
64 Adelaide Grove, London, W12 0JL

Foreword

For me it is a particular pleasure to write a Foreword to this second edition. During my three years of responsibility for the NHS, I suppose a third of my time must have been involved in the questions of the best way of financing our system of health care. This meant the struggle for growth in total resources at a time of economic stringency, the fairest method of distributing available resources, the evolution of effective means of financial controls and of ensuring value for money when the demand outstrips the supply.

Obviously organisations, management structures and manpower are (and always will be) part of the equation.

'Health Service Finance' is an extremely good book by any standard. Concise and well written it is a text book in the sense that it takes the reader systematically through the whole spectrum of organisation, re-organisation, financial planning, allocations and accountability. Yet it is also a 'good read' since it examines alternative methods of financing the NHS into the realms of speculations, augmentations and even political controversy.

Mr H.R. Allan past chairman of the Association of Health Service Treasurers in his foreword to the First Edition in March 1982 wrote 'One can now hope for a long period of stability so that this book may continue as a standard book of reference on NHS Finance for many years to come'.

In fact there have been many changes since 1982: the consolidation of the increased authority of the DHAs, a further squeeze on total resources with the consequently increased difficulty in implementing RAWP in a virtually no growth situation, 'efficiency savings,' Griffiths management scheme and the new relationship with Family Practitioners Committees, to name just a few.

So I warmly welcome the second edition, indicating not only the success of the first edition but giving a chance to reflect some of these changes. But like Mr Allan my plea most strongly is for a period of stability. Too many changes are not good for the service. They also make life more difficult for the student.

Rt. Hon. Lord Ennals
Former Secretary of State for Social Services (1976-79)

Foreword to First Edition

It is with both pleasure and enthusiasm that I welcome the publication of this book on NHS Finance.

Since 1948 there have been many excellent publications, mainly by the Association of Health Service Treasurers and the Chartered Institute of Public Finance and Accountancy, which have dealt with particular aspects of NHS financial matters. This book, however, is the first published since 1951 which has attempted to cover the whole spectrum of NHS finance on the basis of an 'introductory package'.

The book will be useful not only to the student for examination purposes but also as an *aide memoire* to health service accountants. It will also provide a valuable aid to the lay member who wishes to gain a comprehensive insight into the way the NHS manages its financial affairs.

Some of the authors' views are controversial and will not be universally acceptable throughout the NHS but this in no way detracts from the book's value as a standard text book and helps to ensure the reader's interest is sustained.

The timing of publication is particularly opportune as it has enabled the authors to incorporate all the changes introduced on the recent reorganisation of the service. One can now only hope for a long period of stability so that this book may continue to serve as a standard book of reference on NHS Finance for many years to come.

H.R.Allen, BA(Admin), IPFA   *Chairman of the Association*
                                    of Health Service Treasurers March 1982

Contents

List of Tables

List of Figures

List of Abbreviations

AGRA	Advisory Group on Resource Allocation
C & AG	Comptroller and Auditor General
CASPE	Clinical Accountability Service Planning and Evaluation
CBA	Cost Benefit Analysis
CHC	Community Health Council
CIPFA	Chartered Institute of Public Finance and Accountancy
CPRS	Central Policy Review Staff
DCF	Discounted Cash Flow
DGH	District General Hospital
DHA	District Health Authority
DHSS	Department of Health & Social Security
DMT	District Management Team
DRG	Diagnostic Related Group
EEC	European Economic Community
ENT	Ear Nose and Throat
EMT	Extra-territorially Managed
FPC	Family Practitioner Committee
FIS	Financial Information System
GDP	Gross Domestic Product
GP	General Practitioner
HC	Health Circular
HM	Her Majesty's
HMSO	Her Majesty's Stationery Office
HN	Health Notice
HSPI	Health Services Prices Index
HSSB	Health Service Supervisory Board
IRIS	Interactive Resource Information System
NAHA	National Association of Health Authorities
NHS	National Health Service
NO	Nursing Officer
NPV	Net Present Value
PACT	Planning Agreements with Clinical Teams
PB	Programme Budgeting
PBB	Priority Base Budgeting
PESC	Public Expenditure Survey Committee
PI	Performance Indicator
PSBR	Public Sector Borrowing Requirement

RAWP	Resource Allocation Working Party
RCCS	Revenue Consequences of Capital Schemes
RCMA	Revenue Consequences of Medical Appointments
RHA	Regional Health Authority
RT	Regional Treasurer
SAS	Standard Accounting System
SCRAW	Steering Committee on Resource Allocation in Wales
SDP	Social Democratic Party
SFR	Standardised Fertility Ratio
SHARE	Scottish Health Authorities Revenue Equalisation
SIFT	Service Increment for Teaching
SMR	Standardised Mortality ratio
SRSAG	Super Regional Services Advisory Group
TDR	Test Discount Rate
TV	Television
UMG	Unit Management Group
US	United States
USA	United States of America
UWO	Unit Works Officer
VAT	Value Added Tax
VFM	Value for Money
ZBB	Zero Base Budgeting

Preface

Since the first edition of this book was published in 1982 a number of significant developments have occurred which affect the finance and financial management of the NHS. Following the success of the first edition we have been encouraged by a number of people to rewrite the book to take into account such developments. Consequently the second edition takes into account any changes which were publicly announced up to the end of July 1984.

In rewriting the book we have also taken the opportunity to extend it in a number of ways. Firstly we have added brief commentaries on NHS finance in Wales and Scotland. These are not meant to be exhaustive discussions on the subject matter but merely point out the differences between England and the other parts of the United Kingdom. Secondly, we have extended the discussion on alternative ways of financing the NHS and have included an extra chapter on the topic of improving efficiency. It is to be hoped that this will provide a more complete book.

None of this would have been achieved without Jane Gardiner and her typing skills coupled with her ability to decipher illegible manuscripts.

Finally, we wish to thank Rt. Hon. Lord Ennals for writing the Foreword to the second edition, and in particular for his observations on the effect of change on the NHS. His perspectives as a former Secretary of State for Social Services provide a valuable commentary on current developments.

Tom Jones   *October 1984*
Malcolm Prowle

Preface to First Edition

This book has been produced to meet the need for a comprehensive guide to the various aspects of finance in the National Health Service. It has been written in the context of the 1982 reorganisation of the NHS in England and deals with any changes in financial matters consequent on that reorganisation.

The book is divided into four parts. The first part is introductory in nature and discusses the background to the 1982 reorganisation of the NHS in England and its broad consequences. The second part is concerned with the interface between Government and the NHS and considers the procedures for providing funds to the NHS together with a description of how Government influences the planning and control of the use of those funds. The third part of the book focuses, primarily on the new District Health Authorities (DHAs) and discusses resource allocation, planning and control in that context. Finally, the fourth part considers alternative ways in which the NHS might be financed.

This book has been designed to meet the needs of those studying public sector accounting and finance for the examination of:

The Association of Certified Accountants
The Chartered Institute of Public Finance and Accountancy
The Institute of Health Service Administrators

It should also prove useful to students following courses which require a knowledge of public sector finance, such as: The Diploma in Management Studies, The Diploma in Health Service Administration and various degree courses.

Members, officers and clinicians of health authorities who require an authoritative guide to the complexities of NHS Finance should also find it of great use.

Our special thanks must go to Mr Jim Waits, Treasurer of Worcester and District Health Authority and President of the Certified Accountants Health Service Society. Mr Waits has spent countless hours reading through the numerous drafts of this book and offering much constructive criticism and advice. In a real sense, he is very much the third author of this book. However, we hasten to add that all the views expressed are our own. Finally, we wish to thank Mr Roy Allan, Chairman of the Association of Health Service Treasurers, for writing the foreword.

Tom Jones   *October 1981*
Malcolm Prowle

1

Structure of the National Health Service

1.1 Scope

Every organisation has its own specific approach to managing its financial affairs. The particular style, techniques and systems available depend largely on two major factors:

(a) the structure of the organisation
(b) the financial information required by each component of the organisation.

The structure of the NHS was established by the Health Services Act 1980, and was introduced in 1982. The Secretary of State for Social Services is responsible for the NHS in England while in Scotland and Wales the Secretary of State for the appropriate province is responsible. These Ministers are directly accountable to Parliament but look to statutory health authorities and boards to fulfil their duties. These bodies have a constitution and membership which is governed by legislation, the members being appointed rather than elected.

1.2 NHS Structure

In England there are 192 district health authorities (DHAs). These DHAs are accountable to the Secretary of State through 14 regional health authorities (RHAs) for the provision of hospital and community health services. In addition there are a small number of special health authorities and boards of governors which are directly accountable to the Secretary of State for the services provided by highly specialised hospitals and postgraduate teaching hospitals. Services provided by family practitioners such as dentists, opticians and GPs are the responsibility of family practitioner committees (FPCs). At the time of writing, the precise arrangements for FPCs are not yet firm, but there may be some 90 FPCs and clearly in many parts of England the FPC covers an area of more than one DHA. Figure 1 shows the outline structure in England.

Figure 1 – NHS Structure in England

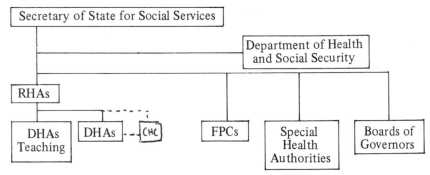

The DHAs provide the vast majority of services and have certain attributes which are important determinants of their financial management. They are all intended to be close to the local community even though they are not accountable to it. While populations of DHAs range from under 100,000 to more than 800,000, closeness is defined more in terms of social geography as served by district general hospitals (DGH).

As one may expect, wide population ranges are also accompanied by a wide range of available financial resources. At the extremes, the smaller DHAs may not receive monies much in excess of £20,000,000 per annum, while at the other end of the scale, the larger DHAs have annual resources in excess of £100,000,000. While many DHAs tend towards the £30,000,000 to £50,000 000 range it is clear that the NHS is comprised of DHAs which have quite different financial characteristics and which therefore may adopt varying approaches to financial management.

DHA size can have significant implications for the methods of resource allocation. RHAs rely considerably on statistical data to assess DHAs needs for resources and in many RHAs this is a version of the formula and approach devised by the Resource Allocation Working Party (RAWP). This is described in Chapters 3 and 6, but briefly, population, demographic, health and cost indicators are combined for each DHA in order to establish the appropriate share of resources that they should receive. While this approach may have been suitable within regions before 1982 when health authorities were generally larger it is reasonable to ask if the approach is still justified without significant modification when applied to generally smaller DHAs. This point is discussed further in Chapter 6.

Another matter related to size is joint planning and finance. Many county and metropolitan district councils now have to collaborate with more than one DHA in the planning and provision of social and health services. In such circumstances it may prove difficult for the agencies involved to reach a common agreement on policy and priorities, leaving them in some difficulty as to the management of services where a joint interest is important. In addition such difficulties may adversely affect the way in which joint finance monies are used. Lack of coterminosity of boundaries will be greater with smaller DHAs and they will therefore tend to be affected by this problem more than the larger DHAs which often share a coterminous boundary with the local authority.

The other main part of the NHS is the family practitioner service. As previously mentioned, at the time of writing, their management arrangements are not yet clear. While the government has stated its intention to supervise these services through FPCs as independant statutory bodies, the current debate also surrounds the way in which they are managed financially. Currently, family practitioner services are provided by general and dental practitioners and opticians who are independent contractors and not subject to cash limits. If cash limits are introduced, it will clearly be a significant development which will be the first step towards the financial control of GPs, dentists and opticians who were previously not constrained by costs or financial considerations when treating patients. While some may argue that they should enjoy such freedom, it is clearly inconsistent for hospital and community health services provided by DHAs to be constrained by cash limits but for family practitioner services provided by contractors to the FPCs to be unrestrained financially. The scope for introducing cash limits for family practitioner services has been examined by a firm of management consultants. Their report is not available at the time of writing and we await the outcome with interest.

One public body not shown on figure 1 is the community health council (CHC). It is excluded from the table because it does not provide services but can be thought of as the consumer's watchdog. A CHC exists for each DHA and is financed by a cash limit fixed by the RHA. While expenditure on CHCs appears in the DHAs accounts and is counted against the DHAs management cost ceiling, it is important to understand that CHCs are independent of DHAs.

The NHS management arrangements have recently been examined

by a team of businessmen, the NHS Management Inquiry or Griffiths Inquiry, which concluded that the overall management of the NHS could be improved. Two of its recommendations were that a Health Services Supervisory Board (HSSB) and a NHS Management Board should be established. The HSSB would be chaired by the Secretary of State. Other members would include the Minister of State (Health), the Permanent Secretary and the Chief Medical Officer, and would deal with the overall objectives, strategic issues, resource allocation and performance of the NHS. The NHS Management Board would take responsibility for all the existing NHS management responsibilities in the DHSS. The Griffiths Report envisages that the Chairman would be drawn from outside the NHS and have two particular roles; the Secretary of States "right hand man" and the Accounting Officer for NHS expenditure.

Changes to the management arrangements within health authorities are also being considered. Rather than the concensus approach, Griffiths recommends the appointment of a general manager at both the RHA and DHA level and for each unit of management within a DHA. The authority's general manager could be one of the existing chief officers or a separate appointment, perhaps for a limited period. The post would remove the general management responsibilities from the existing chief officers leaving them with their specific responsibilities.

These proposals were published in October 1983. At the time of writing their implementation is imminent.

1.3   DHA Management Structure

The main document governing DHA management structure is HC(80)8. This laid down a requirement on each DHA to appoint a district management team (DMT) and to subdivide its services into appropriate units which would then be managed by a unit management group (UMG). The roles and membership of the DMT and UMGs are quite separate and distinct.

The DMT has six members as follows:

Chief Officers:

(a) District Administrator
(b) District Medical Officer
(c) District Nursing Officer
(d) District Treasurer

Medical Representatives:

(e) Consultant
(f) General Practitioner

This excludes the effect of Griffiths' proposals.

The four chief officers are individually accountable to the DHA for their own sphere of responsibility as well as being jointly responsible as the DMT for the management and planning of services. This shared responsibility leads to the concept of consensus management which requires the DMT to attempt to reach an agreed position on issues such as management policy and advice to the DHA on service priorities both in the short and long term. Clearly on matters of such magnitude consensus does not mean seeking unanimity at all costs. Where members on the DMT cannot reach agreement without compromising their specific responsibilities then such significant differences would comprised real choices for the DHA.

This consensus approach has been examined against the chief executive style, by the Griffiths Inquiry, which has recommended that an overall general manager be appointed. Two important features of this alternative style are worth noting. In our opinion, decisions taken by a chief executive will still require the support of the DMT members if they are to succeed and in this respect the approach may prove to be no different to the consensus style. Secondly, it is important that any significant differences of view of DMT members are made known to the DHA when major issues are being considered. This will help to provide real choices and improve policy making compared to a system which provides an opportunity for the chief executive to filter such differences and stifle debate in the public forum of the DHA.

UMGs operate at a structural level which is subordinate to the DMT. They manage discrete and identifiable service groups such as a DGH, psychiatric services or community services. The membership of UMGs can vary between DHAs, but as a minimum should include the unit administrator, a director of nursing services and a representative of the medical profession. Some DHAs include a Treasurers' representative on the UMG, others adopt the approach where the Treasurers' representative attends and provides financial advice without actually being a member of the UMG. Similarly in some DHAs a unit works officer (UWO) is also a member of the unit management team.

The various approaches to providing financial advice to a UMG may well have arisen because UMGs are not necessarily expected to reach agreement on solutions to management problems and issues. In this respect it is not critical to successful management for Treasurers representatives to be full members. However, it is critical that they participate in UMG activities in order to ensure that decisions are taken in the knowledge and understanding of the financial implications.

While there is no requirement on UMGs to reach consensus in decision making, a specific relationship exists between the UMG members. The unit administrator not only controls the budgets for which he is directly responsible but also co-ordinates other unit budgets. It can be seen that the unit budget and the unit administrator are key elements in a health authority's financial management arrangements. With a large degree of delegation to UMGs, the way in which the unit budget is managed will clearly affect the financial performance of the authority. It is therefore imperative that unit budgets are managed with a high degree of involvement of Treasurer's staff and within clear and sound policies of virement. This will ensure consistency between UMGs and help to prevent unwise budgetary adjustments. In this context the Treasurer's role can be seen as being one of a central overview with the interest of the Authority, rather than any particular UMG, being paramount. Again the Griffiths Inquiry team has recommended that a general manager is appointed for each unit.

1.4   The Role of the District Treasurer

One important issue for the District Treasurer is his relationship with the general manager and how this links with their specific responsibilities. On financial matters this distinction may not always be clear cut but it is critical that a delineation is agreed by those responsible in health authorities. This has been observed elsewhere. In particular the Royal Commission on the NHS commented that 'consensus management may sap individual responsibility by allowing it to be shared'. HC(80)8 reminded DHAs and DMT members of the distinction between the types of responsibilities and the dangers arising from any misunderstandings. This was highlighted by the Management Inquiry.

Most of the Treasurers individual responsibilities are described by the Financial Directors for Health Authorities in England. It is made explicit that the Treasurer is the provider of financial information to budgetholders and that monitoring budgets is a specific responsibility of the Treasurer.

Other tasks include the provision of an internal audit service, the prescription of accounting procedures to ensure sound financial control and the preparation of budgets and estimates.

One duty stands out above all others as having special significance, namely the provision of financial advice to the authority and its officers. This is particularly important in its relationship between the Treasurer and the general manager. At the time of writing, it seems likely that the general manager will be required to implement the DHAs financial policies after taking account of advice given by the Treasurer. While the Treasurer has specific responsibility as the financial advisor to the DHA and general management, other DMT members should be as interested as the Treasurer in financial issues.

One other important task in which the Treasurer has a major responsibility is in the implementation and use of investment appraisal. While this is not referred to specifically in the financial directors the ~~tions~~ Treasurer will wish to ensure that decisions in relation to the spending and saving of money are taken wisely and with full knowledge of the effects both financially and in relation to patients. The Treasurer's interest in investment appraisal is a natural part of his role as the Authority's financial adviser.

A major aspect of the Treasurer's responsibility is his participation with all other members of the DMT in decisions relating to standards and levels of services. This would include matters such as medical and nurse staffing levels, service developments, service reductions and monitoring of services. The Treasurer's involvement in such matters can be clearly justified as a natural part of the consensus approach adopted for the formulation of financial policy. Even with a general manager directly responsible for levels and quality of service we still see a need for all Chief Officers to develop and share a common understanding of policy issues.

1.5 NHS Structure in Scotland and Wales

The arrangements in Scotland and Wales differ from England in that RHAs do not feature. The authorities or boards are accountable directly to the appropriate Secretary of State. In addition there are certain distinguishing characteristics, the main one being that in Wales the DHAs were based on the former Area Health Authority rather than the districts as in most of England. Scotland could be similar to Wales if reports at the time of writing are correct. This arrangement leads to larger health authorities with more UMGs than is generally the case in England. While boards are to be found in Scotland and authorities in Wales, their structures are alike. They all cover relatively large geographic units and the membership of the management teams are similar. The management team structures are in fact similar to the arrangements for English DHAs and in this respect a similar approach to financial management could be predicted.

2

Financing the
National Health Service

2.1 The Government's Contribution

Unlike the health services of many other developed countries the NHS
is financed almost entirely from the Government's National Exchequer.
This is illustrated in Table 1 which shows the composition of NHS
finance for 1982/83.

Table 1– NHS Financing in 1982/83 for Great Britain

Source of Finance	£m	%
National Exchequer	12,513	86
National Insurance Fund	1,600	11
Other Sources	436	3
Total Expenditure in Great Britain	14,549	100

Although the amount financed from 'other sources' is not large in
total, its importance varies between health authorities. Income from
patients' represents about 90% of the other income. The possibility of
increasing and extending the range of charges will be considered in
Chapter 9 along with extended insurance arrangements.

The contribution of 86% is a general appropriation from the National
Exchequer. Consequently, it must compete for scarce resources with
other Government programmes such as defence and education. This
general appropriation is contrary to the belief held by some people that
the NHS is financed entirely from National Insurance contributions.
This is clearly not so, but such a method of finance is a possible
alternative which we have considered in Chapter 9.

This analysis can be subdivided further by comparing the gross
expenditure in the three countries.

Table 2 – NHS Expenditure in 1982/83 for Great Britain

	£m	%
England	12,134	84
Scotland	1,648	11
Wales	767	5
Total Expenditure in Great Britain	14,549	100

Initially we have outlined the main source of NHS finance, namely the Government's contribution together with the geographic distribution of expenditure. This necessarily leads us to the question: *How is the total allocation of Government finance arrived at?*

2.2   Influences on the Allocation of Funds to Government Programmes

It seems to us that the allocation of funds to the various Government programmes could be described as a politico-economic process. In the first instance the Government must decide on the total level of public expenditure that it believes it can undertake. In the past, and especially during the 1970's, this seemed to have been largely determined by a consideration of the economic state of the nation. If the economy was buoyant, as measured in terms of economic parameters such as growth and unemployment, then a higher level of public expenditure was possible than if the economy was in decline.

The present Conservative Government, following a broadly monetarist approach, argues that a reduction in the level of public expenditure will enable them to reduce the Public Sector Borrowing Requirement (PSBR). It is hoped that the reduced PSBR coupled with other policies will lead to a reduction in the rate of inflation, this being the prime economic objective of the Government. The Labour party in Opposition together with the SDP/Liberal Alliance, follow a neo-Keynsian approach, and advocate the stimulation of aggregate demand coupled with increases in the level of public expenditure, with the intention of reducing the level of unemployment. This is clearly a simplification of the economic policies of the political parties, but it does seem that there is no consistent posture as regards the level of public expenditure.

Once the total level of planned public spending has been settled, the Government can consider its allocation to the various programmes. The factors affecting this allocation are complex but we suggest that the major influence is political. Different Governments with different social and political views will give greater emphasis to some programmes than to others. It is worth noting that some writers have also suggested that an important factor in the allocation of public expenditure is the personality of the individual Minister and his political 'clout', but this analysis is open to question.

These political views prevail in the process of planning levels of public spending. In recent years successive Governments have used a similar mechanism to express their own particular preferences for public spending.

2.3 The Decision Making Process

The procedures are rather complex and are cyclical in nature but we shall attempt to explain what happens over the course of one financial year and as our starting point we shall consider the work of the Public Expenditure Survey Committee (PESC).

Following the report of the Plowden Committee in 1961, the PESC was created to assist in the planning of public expenditure. This committee comprises senior civil servants from government spending departments and is chaired by a senior Treasury official. It is intended to provide a searching examination of the Government's expenditure plans for the ensuing years in an attempt to identify priorities. In response to instructions from HM Treasury, government departments submit to the Treasury detailed estimates of their future expenditure. These plans are then scrutinised by the PESC and the net result of its deliberations is the preparation of a report for the Chancellor of the Exchequer, who then presents this report to the Cabinet. Over the summer and autumn months, the Cabinet will deliberate over the contents of the PESC report in an attempt to reach a decision about the total amount and allocation of public expenditure. Such a decision will be based not only on the context of the PESC report but also on other factors such as the financial and economic outlook, social policies of the Government and political judgement. During the Autumn the Chancellor of the Exchequer will make an economic statement outlining the main aspects of future public spending. In the following spring the Cabinet's decision over public expenditure will be made public through the publication of a White Paper on Public Expenditure. These White Papers show details of public expenditure, by programme, for the following periods:

(a) previous years
(b) estimated outturn for current year
(c) plans for future years.

Other additional information is shown in the White Paper, including:

(a) the nature of the expenditure – capital or current
(b) the spending body – such as central government, local government, nationalised industry.

Table 3 summarises the Government's expenditure programmes for the period 1983/84 to 1985/86.

The expenditure programmes adopt the concept of cash planning. This requires assumptions to be made about pay and price increases in the current and future years of the programme. In this way the Government can forecast the amount of cash it intends to spend and then use this figure to estimate its various targets such as total public expenditure, taxation levels and public sector borrowing requirement.

Including estimated inflation in the expenditure plans usually results in planned NHS expenditure showing an increase, and it is important to distinguish inflationary increases from real growth. The latter is additional money over and above that required to pay for inflation and because of the uncertainties about inflation predictions the programmes are not clear statements about which services will grow and which will contract. This problem can be exacerbated by the tendency of Governments to underestimate inflation assumptions in order to present an optimistic view of the future performance of the economy. In addition, the inflation assumptions tend to be modified when the particular year arrives and becomes subject to the cash limit procedure. Public Expenditure White Papers using this cash planning base tend therefore to be of relatively limited value as detailed statements of Government policy on particular services such as the NHS. The previous methodology used constant prices which excluded inflation assumptions, and this approach did not have the problems of identifying growth associated with cash planning.

It is important to realise that this White Paper is a planning document showing an outline of the Government's intentions and aspirations for public expenditure within a view of the anticipated economic performance of the country. It is not a control device. Much of public expenditure is outside the control of Government, being determined independently by, for example, local authorities and nationalised industries. In reality, the authority to incur Government spending must first be given by Parliament via the Parliamentary Estimates procedure. This is the control device for Government spending, including that on the NHS, and follows on from the PESC process.

1983/84 to 1985/86 - Source Cmnd 8789

	1977-78 outturn £ million	1978-79 outturn £ million	1979-80 outturn £ million	1980-81 outturn £ million	1981-82 outturn £ million	1982-83 estimated outturn £ million	1983-84 plans £ million	1984-85 plans £ million	1985-86 plans £ million
Defence	6,821	7,496	9,227	11,180	12,606	14,411	15,987	17,290	18,330
Overseas aid and other overseas services									
Overseas aid	599	723	788	888	960	959	1,057	1,100	1,130
Net payments to EC institutions	542	751	839	221	153	580	380	450	530
Other overseas services	426	378	454	515	573	663	737	770	800
Agriculture, fisheries, food and forestry	866	813	1,007	1,347	1,372	1,784	1,754	1,650	1,730
Industry, energy, trade and employment	2,233	3,036	2,881	4,011	5,319	5,854	5,622	5,490	5,410
Transport	2,270	2,447	2,966	3,456	3,898	4,340	4,302	4,530	4,690
Housing	3,418	3,572	4,514	4,457	3,137	2,579	2,792	2,990	3,110
Other environmental services	1,955	2,257	2,702	3,231	3,244	3,433	3,564	3,680	3,800
Law, order and protective services	1,791	2,036	2,579	3,167	3,774	4,284	4,583	4,820	5,040
Education and science	7,039	7,755	8,946	10,901	11,828	12,628	12,560	12,910	13,340
Arts and libraries	299	340	404	477	520	579	563	580	600
Health and personal social services	6,542	7,425	8,899	11,362	12,751	13,879	14,608	15,380	16,070
Social security	13,917	16,437	19,417	23,458	28,510	32,473	34,394	35,940	37,900
Other public services	912	969	1,159	1,439	1,556	1,670	1,675	1,740	1,830
Common services	766	853	1,009	1,099	1,453	1,652	997	1,080	1,190
Scotland	3,234	3,683	4,447	5,324	5,772	6,263	6,384	6,580	6,790
Wales	1,279	1,477	1,790	2,129	2,243	2,379	2,528	2,610	2,720
Northern Ireland	1,816	2,137	2,452	2,905	3,218	3,568	3,806	4,020	4,210
Government lending to nationalised industries	-205	705	1,941	2,222	1,457	1,363	1,113	1,250	940
Local authority current expenditure not allocated to programmes (England)							904	460	250
Adjustments									
Public corporations' net overseas and market borrowing	817	443	-481	-617	260	-1,085	-292	-440	-660
Special sales of assets	-548		-999	-356	79	-550	-750	-1,500	-500
Contingency reserve						250	1,500		
Provisional reserves								3,000	3,000
General allowance for shortfall						-950	-1,200		
Planning Total	56,789	65,734	76,939	92,815	104,684	113,007	119,568	126,370	132,260

In the Spring prior to the commencement of a particular financial year, money is voted by Parliament in the Main Estimates. This voting procedure is the legal authorisation for the Government to spend. The amounts voted are based on the relevant year of the White Paper with minor modifications, either increases or reductions.

The year 1976/77 heralded the introduction of cash limits on all items of public expenditure which were not demand based. Therefore, the NHS is subject to cash limits, but the spending of FPCs is not. Under the cash limit procedures a predetermined limit is placed on the amount that the Treasury is prepared to request from Parliament, to cover inflation in pay and prices to the end of the financial year. This upper limit is fixed and will not normally be altered if actual inflation exceeds it.

The cash limit system is complex and more will be said about it in Chapters 5 & 6. Figure 2 illustrates the public expenditure review process for a typical year, using 1984/85 as an example.

Figure 2 – Planning of Public Spending 1984/85

Timing	*Event*
Winter 1982/83	Treasury issues survey guidelines and spending departments develop plans.
Spring 1983	Treasury discusses plans with spending departments and PESC Report prepared.
Summer 1983	PESC Report circulated with Treasury and spending departments and Cabinet considers Treasury's preliminary assessment of spending projections.
Autumn 1983	Treasury and spending Ministers discuss details and reach agreements on spending levels and unresolved issues finalised by Cabinet.
	Chancellor of the Exchequer reports outline programme to Parliament, usually in November.
Winter 1983/84	White Paper on Public Expenditure published usually in February.
Spring 1984	Parliamentary Estimates for 1984/85 approved and cash limits issued usually in March. Financial year 1984/85 begins on 1st April 1984.
Spring 1985	Financial year 1984/85 ends on 31st March 1985.

2.4 Family Practitioner Committees (FPCs)

NHS finance has two major components:

(a) that part which is cash limited and relates to services provided by health authorities.
(b) that part which is not cash limited and relates to the FPCs, for services provided by GPs, dental practitioners and opticians contracted to FPCs.

The level of spending on family practitioner services is determined by the demand placed upon them by the users. Thus the level of spending is related directly to the number of GPs, dentists and opticians paid and the number of patients treated by them. In England these FPCs are due to become independent statutory authorities.

While the total spending is not controlled, the sum required each year can be estimated reasonably well and financial provision is made centrally in DHSS budgets. The distribution of these resources, however, is not the subject of resource allocation mechanisms to ensure that each locality has its fair share, but is the direct result of the levels of service. This blank cheque treatment of FPC finance makes the whole process so simple that we have not considered the matter later in the book but have mentioned it here for completeness.

The income attributable to the FPC is that arising from prescription charges on GPs prescriptions, charges for dental treatment and for the supply of spectacles and optical appliances. The levels of charge are determined by the Secretary of State as are the exemptions from such charges, for example, for children and older members of the population.

The aspect of FPC finance which requires particular comment is the lack of a cash limit. Recently a firm of management consultants were commissioned by the Secretary of State to examine the feasibility of introducing cash limits into the FPC. Their report was submitted but has never been presented to the NHS for consideration. We can only assume because of the lack of any change that the report was shelved because it either supported the present system or proved to be so radical that it would have produced the inevitable financial constraint on practitioners which would have been unacceptable to the professionals. A simply financed open ended FPC seems to be with us for the foreseeable future.

2.5   Changes in the Levels of NHS Finance

Recently, public debate about the level of NHS finance has been extensive. To some extent this may be attributed to the introduction of cash planning which tends to combine and thus confuse inflationary increases and real growth. One major contribution to the debate was the publication of *Health Care and Its Costs* by HMSO.

This revealed that over the ten years 1972 to 1982 the resources available to the NHS had increased. Two measures used were the share of national gross domestic product for the NHS, which increased from 4% to 5½% over the ten years, and the real increase in resources of 23% over the same period. It is interesting to note that this increase was fairly steady over the period and could be attributed to all Governments during the period.

Since the end of that ten year period in March 1982 the resource picture has changed, with 1983/84 in particular seeing a significant financial adjustment when the Chancellor of the Exchequer persuaded the Government to reduce the cash for health authorities by some 1% in July 1983. This was seen as necessary in order to finance an unexpected increase in spending by the FPCs. The effect was to wipe out the health authorities growth for the year. However, his economic statement in November of the same year saw the 1% reinstated for 1984/85 but the prospect for additional growth was limited. This can be compared with the Secretary of State's planned average level of increase of ½% per annum over the ten years 1984/85 to 1993/94.

2.6   Scotland and Wales

Spending plans for health services in Scotland and Wales are not included in the White Paper's general category of health and personal social services. Instead, they are grouped under the total planned public expenditure for those two parts of the Country which are shown separately in the White Paper. In this respect the plans for Scotland and Wales are in essence prepared by using their own PESC cycles, and the respective Secretary's of State can determine how much of their programme will be allocated to health services. Obviously discussions with the Treasury and within the Cabinet itself provide an opportunity to achieve a consistency of policy between England, Scotland and Wales where this is desirable.

3

Allocations to Regional Health Authorities

3.1 Types of Allocations

In this chapter, we consider the allocation of resources to RHAs. Resources in this context means money.

There are three categories which are different in nature and require different criteria when making allocations. It is therefore important to understand the distinctions, which we outline as follows:

(a) revenue – the money required to finance the day to day spending of health services. For example, it is used to pay the salaries and wages of employees.
(b) capital – the money required to finance the acquisition of assets. For example, it is used to pay for the building of new hospitals.
(c) earmarked allocations – these are allocations for specified purposes: for example, joint financing of projects with local authorities. The allocation may be capital or revenue or both.

3.2 Revenue Allocations to RHAs – the General Aims

Before outlining the present revenue allocation procedures and some possible alternatives, we shall first discuss some general principles underlying resource allocation and consider why earlier methods of allocating funds to RHAs are now considered to be inappropriate. The NHS as its name suggests is a *national* service thus implying the same or similar standards of service in all parts of the country. In 1945, Aneurin Bevan, later to become the first Minister of Health, said 'We have got to achieve as nearly as possible a uniform standard of service for all'. This indicates to us the first general principle of resource allocation: equity – resources must be distributed among health authorities in such a way as to ensure equal access to health services for all persons at equal risk, wherever they may live.

The second principle of resource allocation appears, to us, to be objectivity. By this we mean that given a particular method of resource allocation it would be possible for any number of persons to arrive at a similar distribution of funds between health authorities. It is not necessary for these persons to agree that the method of allocation is the best one, only that given the method, they can achieve a consensus.

The third general principle could be termed simplicity. It is desirable that the method of resource allocation be simple enough to be understood by most of the people affected by it and furthermore that the resource allocation procedures themselves are not time-consuming and hence expensive to operate.

Clearly no perfect method of resource allocation is possible and various compromises will have to be made between these general principles.

When we come to consider resource allocation in practice, we find a somewhat surprising situation. In spite of the emphasis on the national aspects of the NHS, with its ideals of a uniform standard of service and equal access to health services for all, evidence suggests that there are substantial inequalities in the distribution of resources between different parts of England and that these inequalities have persisted since the establishment of the NHS on 5th July 1948. Although we accept that inequalities in the distribution of resources does not automatically imply inequalities in the standard of health services, the inequality of resources is such that it seems reasonable to assume that standards of service will vary between different parts of the country. It is somewhat ironic that despite this emphasis on the national aspects of the NHS, there exist less inequalities in, for example, the education service which is administered by autonomous local authorities working under central government guidance.

The persistance of such inequalities has been described as being the result of a combination of policy-inertia and demographic drag. This implies a criticism of resource allocation procedures applied during the first twenty five years of the NHS's life whereby allocations, each year, to health authorities were based primarily on the allocation it received in the previous year and the need to finance the revenue costs of any completed capital schemes. It took no account of any demographic factors or changes and thus the initial inequalities in the resources available to health authorities have been perpetuated. These inequalities can crudely be described as resulting in relatively more resources for RHAs in South East England at the expense of the rest of the country. In reality, the situation is more complex than this, as it is possible to find large inequalities in resources available to the DHAs within each region. The existence of such inequalities appears to be inconsistent with the idea of a *national* health service, and is now unacceptable to all governments. We shall now look at some of the attempts made in recent years to rectify the situation.

3.3 The Crossman Formula

The first attempt came in the early 1970s on the initiative of the then Secretary of State, the late Richard Crossman. This method of resource allocation utilised a formula which is now referred to as the Crossman formula. Revenue funds were to be distributed to regions on the basis of such factors as population served; beds provided; cases dealt with. It was intended that the inequalities would be eradicated over a 10-year period. However, in spite of its revolutionary nature, the Crossman formula failed. Three years after its introduction the relative inequality between regions was virtually unchanged. It appears that the lack of success of this approach was due to the pre-empting of additional revenue monies for two particular purposes:

(a) Revenue consequences of capital schemes (RCCS) – a system under which the DHSS set aside additional revenue to finance the running costs of new developments.
(b) The guarantee that each hospital board would receive at least ¼% annual growth in revenue in addition to any RCCS.

The pre-empting of funds for these two purposes meant that very little additional money was available to eradicate relative inequalities. This was accompanied by a reluctance to redistribute the existing revenue allocations between hospital boards and hence the inequalities persisted.

3.4 The Resource Allocation Working Party (RAWP)

Clearly, a new approach to the problem was needed and in 1975 the then Secretary of State appointed the RAWP. As its terms of reference, it had to review the arrangements for distributing capital and revenue to health authorities, with a view to establishing a method of securing a pattern of distribution which would be responsive to relative need. The method was expected to be objective, equitable and efficient. It is important to note that the RAWP was not asked to comment on the adequacy of the total resources availabe to the NHS, nor was it to concern itself with how the funds allocated to health authorities were to be deployed. The RAWP was only to concern itself with how a given amount of money might be distributed between health authorities. The recommendations of the RAWP were published in 1976, and now dominate the subject and method of resource allocation in the NHS, so we have outlined the conclusions of the RAWP and the recommendations they made. Most of these have now been implemented.

Funds voted by Parliament for health authorities must find their way down the NHS structure to the DHAs. This allocation procedure is in fact a binary process. A primary allocation is made from the DHSS to RHAs and a secondary allocation made from RHAs to DHAs. Although there are common features to both primary and secondary allocations, and indeed the RAWP report itself commented on both types, in this chapter we have concentrated on the RAWP recommendations as they affect the distribution of funds between RHAs. This we have called inter-regional RAWP. After discussing the methodology of inter-regional RAWP, we shall critically examine this method of allocation bearing in mind the general principles outlined earlier.

3.5   Inter-Regional RAWP

The RAWP report attempted to identify what were termed criteria of need. The need for health services in this context is not absolute but relative, and designed to indicate the relative need for resources across the country. Five main criteria were selected which were regarded as indicative of relative need:

(a) Size of population – as health services are supplied to people, clearly population size must be the primary factor in establishing the relative need for resources.

(b) Population structure – it can easily be demonstrated that different segments of a population have different needs for health services. For example elderly persons need far more health care than their proportionate part of the population would suggest. Again, women have different needs from men, and children too are heavily dependent on health services. Clearly the age/sex structure of the population is important in determining the relative need for resources.

(c) Morbidity, (sickness) – It is self-evident that the greater the level of sickness existing in an area the greater will be the relative need for health services. It can be shown that even when variations in age/sex structure are accounted for, populations of the same size and structure exhibit variations in the level of morbidity. Therefore the levels of morbidity, which can be influenced by a variety of factors such as social and environmental, must also be taken into account.

(d) Cost-weighting – The overall level of morbidity prevailing in a region is determined by the incidence of each of a large number of possible clinical conditions. Available statistical evidence, suggests that the cost of providing health services varies considerably, according to the condition being treated. Consequently, the RAWP recognised that when allocating resources to RHAs, it is necessary to take into account the cost of treating the various clinical conditions occurring in those regions. There is, therefore, a need for information about the costs of treating the different clinical conditions. This could then be reflected in the relative need for resources.

(e) Health services across administrative boundaries – for a number of reasons, the boundaries of health authorities cannot be regarded as sacrosanct. It is common for patients resident in one health authority to obtain treatment in another. These cross-boundary flows, as they are termed, may occur either between RHAs or between DHAs within an RHA. They are mainly the result of two factors. First, the right of doctors to refer patients wherever they, the doctors, wish. Secondly, the fact that few health authorities, especially DHAs, are entirely self-sufficient in terms of service provision. For example, expensive highly specialised treatment for a relatively small number of patients, such as for renal transplants, would be provided by one DHA for the whole region. Clearly, therefore, these cross-boundary flows of patients are also an important factor in determining the relative need for resources and must be taken into account.

Although the RAWP recognised that the above criteria were the important ones in determining relative need they also recognised that there were practical difficulties involved in dealing with some of these factors. Two of the factors, population size and structure, presented few problems. Statistical information is readily available on both of these factors and it is then possible to apply, to the component parts of the population, a weighting to reflect the demand made by each age/sex group on health services.

The third factor, morbidity, presents real problems. In the first instance it is conceptually difficult to measure morbidity in terms of sickness levels. *How does one decide when a person is sick or not or whether one person is more sick than another?* Furthermore, sickness can only be measured when there is some sort of information-capture about it. So for example when a person enters hospital, consults his GP or reports absence from work due to sickness there is some indication of the incidence of morbidity, but if a housewife feeling sick merely stays in the house or a man feeling sick still goes to work there is no information captured. Several possible measures of morbidity were considered by the RAWP, such as waiting lists and case loads, but all were discarded. The RAWP finally decided to recommend the use of mortality statistics (death rates), as a substitute for morbidity. Whether this substitution of mortality for morbidity can be justified we shall discuss later. For the moment, we note the use of regional standardised mortality ratios (SMRs) for each RHA, as surrogates for morbidity in determining the relative need for resources. Standardised fertility ratios (SFRs) were also used to indicate the need for maternity services.

Cost-weightings also caused problems for the simple reason that the required information did not exist and presumably still does not. As will be seen in Chapter 5, financial information systems in the NHS tend to be functionally orientated. For example, costs are analysed by the nursing function and the catering function. These are not geared towards the provision of information about the costs of treating patients for a variety of conditions. A considerable amount of research is currently taking place with the aim of establishing the cost of treating different clinical conditions but currently such a factor is reflected by the use of cost data derived from a multiple regression analysis of hospital cost statements.

Finally we come to the factor concerning health services provided in other RHAs – the so-called cross-boundary flow of patients. To enable these cross-boundary flows to be taken into account when determining the relative need of a particular authority, it is necessary to determine the number of patients 'imported' into the RHA, and the number 'exported' to other RHAs. Fortunately, in the case of hospital in-patients, statistical data on these cross-boundary flows is readily available, mainly via the Hospital Activity Analysis, but for day and out-patients the absence of any reliable statistical information means that little account can be taken of any such cross-boundary flows.

3.6   Applying the Principles

Adopting a pragmatic approach, the RAWP used its own five criteria of relative need and expressed these using the best available information. These RAWP factors are combined to build up an overall measure of relative need for each RHA. This procedure is illustrated in Figure 3.

To compute a RAWP target for each RHA, the RAWP approach was to break down the health services provided into seven different aspects and to treat each of these in a different way. The starting point for each of these was to be a base population. In some cases, such as the ambulance service, the base population was to be the crude mid-year estimated population for the region, while in other cases, such as non psychiatric in-patient services, the

Figure 3 – The Build-Up of a RAWP Target

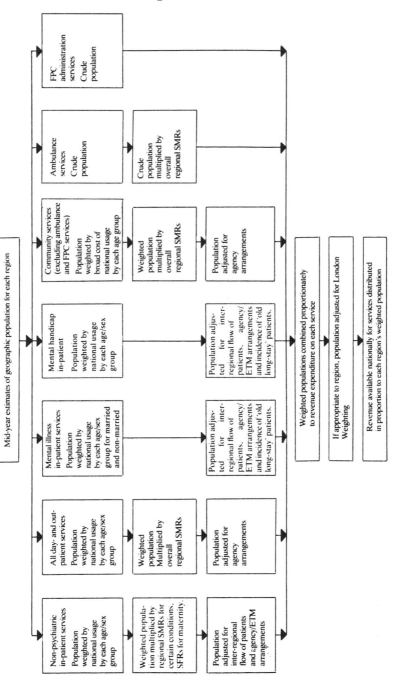

base population was to be the crude population weighted by the national use of the service by each age/sex group. Consequently, a base population was arrived at for each of the seven service-aspects.

The next step was to take account of regional morbidity and this was done by multiplying four of the RAWP populations by the regional SMRs for the relevant service aspects. SFRs were also used for non-psychiatric inpatient services where relevant. No adjustments for mortality were made to the mental illness, mental handicap and FPC administration services as it is not really a relevant factor in these cases. Finally, adjustments are made to five of the RAWP populations to take into account the cross-boundary flow of patients between regions and also agency arrangements between regions.

The seven adjusted RAWP populations for each of the seven service-aspects now have to be combined. This is done by weighting each of these seven populations by a factor which represents the proportion of revenue expenditure spent nationally on that particular service-aspect in the previous year. The seven populations are then summated to give an overall factor for the RHA expressed as a weighted population figure. This procedure is carried out for all RHAs and so the DHSS has a weighted population for each RHA which expresses the relative need for resources in that region.

Taking the national revenue figure for health authorities recommended by the Government to Parliament and approved in the Parliamentary Estimates, the RAWP target for each RHA is then calculated. The target is produced by sharing out this national figure in proportion to the overall weighted populations. It is important to emphasise that the use of these RAWP factors only assists in building up a profile of the *relative* need of RHAs and therefore only indicates the proportion of revenue available nationally that a particular authority *should* receive. In other words it is a target allocation. When the RAWP compared the target allocation for RHAs with the previous years revenue allocation received by them, the degree of inequality between RHAs referred to earlier, became evident. Figure 4 illustrates the point.

Figure 4 shows a clear picture of the four Thames RHAs plus the Oxford RHA receiving more resources than their calculated RAWP target whilst the rest of England, especially the RHAs in the North, is below target. Admittedly, the acceptance of such inequality depends on ones acceptance of the validity of the RAWP formula. While there are some objections to the accuracy of the formula, we would still argue that the RAWP approach is the best available indicator of the distribution of resources and that its findings should be heeded.

In recommending a move towards greater equality of resources, the

Figure 4 – Comparisons of 1977/78 Targets with 1976/77 Allocations

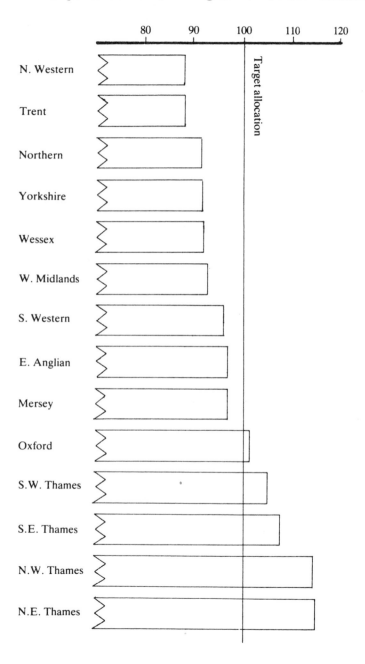

RAWP recognised that there are practical limits to the amount of reduction which any of the over-target RHAs could stand in any one year, especially in view of the need to remedy the relative inequality which exists within the over target RHAs. Conversely there is also a limit to the amount of additional revenue which any RHA could effectively and efficiently absorb in a year. This view was once expressed by a Treasurer in an under-target region with the words: 'We believe that if we were given an extra million pounds we wouldn't know what to do with it'. While this might be an overstatement, it does give some idea of the problem. The RAWP therefore recommended that any re-distribution should be performed gradually over a period of years and that there should be limits to the amount of any reduction in the allocations for over-target RHAs which could be transferred to under-target RHAs. Ceilings and floors were therefore created: ceilings being the maximum percentage growth in resources that any RHA could absorb in any one year and floors being the maximum percentage reduction a RHA could withstand in a year. The level of the ceilings and floors was not to be considered constant but would vary depending on whether the NHS, as a whole, obtained growth or suffered cutback .

As previously mentioned, the recommendations of the RAWP now provide the mechanism for inter-regional resource allocation in the NHS. It might be thought that the major problems of revenue allocations are now ironed out and the RAWP method is fully accepted. However, this is by no means the case and we shall now look at some of the drawbacks and defects of the RAWP approach that have been identified.

3.7   Drawbacks and Defects of the RAWP Targets

The first major defect of the RAWP philosophy is that it is only concerned with the re-distribution of money. Health services are, in fact, provided by people using equipment and buildings. While it is relatively easy to come up with a method for re-distributing money between RHAs it is not so easy to shift these physical resources. For example, specialist doctors may be unwilling to move away from London into the provinces, even though funds are available in the provinces to employ additional clinicians. Furthermore, it is clearly impossible to uproot hospital buildings and shift them to another part of the country and so merely re-allocating funds on the basis of population needs could result in an under-utilisation of present NHS buildings. However, if funds are allocated on the basis of existing employment and building patterns, this merely perpetuates the historical method of provision and regional inequality.

The second defect of the RAWP method of allocation concerns possible defects in the RAWP formula itself. It can be argued that the factors included in the RAWP formula do not, in themselves, satisfactorily measure relative need and so result in a distortion of the allocation process. Some authors have discussed this in detail. The main criticisms can be summarised as follows:

(a) We have already mentioned the absence from the RAWP formula of an adequate weighting factor to reflect the different costs of treating different clinical conditions. On the basis of the limited information available it appears that this could be a significant factor, but until more accurate data is available on the costs of clinical treatment, little more can be said about this.

(b) There exists considerable doubt about the significance of the relationship between morbidity and mortality as measured by regional SMRs. Intuitively, this seems at least partially true as there are a number of clinical complaints such as arthritis which do not necessarily lead to death but the treatment of which does require health service resources. The measurement of true morbidity is a seemingly intractable problem and although there is no satisfactory answer about the link between morbidity and mortality, it should be noted that research work is being undertaken to devise more adequate measures of morbidity.

(c) The absence of a factor to reflect the incidence between regions, of cross-boundary flows of day-patients and out-patients could be a serious defect. For example, it would seem reasonable to assume that the cross-boundary flows of day-patients and out-patients between the London based regions could be of the same order as those of in-patients, which are themselves quite significant. The RAWP report saw an urgent need to assemble better information about this group of patients who attract a substantial and increasing proportion of NHS expenditure. A number of small scale studies of out-patient flows have been carried out by some RHAs since RAWP reported, but a report has suggested that the limited results do not form the basis for making adjustments between those regions and that a large scale study would be required.

(d) The RAWP formula contains no factor to reflect geographic variations in the market cost of obtaining resources. Recent studies have suggested that the cost of obtaining manpower is considerably greater in the Thames regions than other regions in England and that variations occur between the four Thames RHAs themselves. Although a partial compensation for this higher cost is made via the London weighting, it is suggested that this is inadequate and does not reflect the true cost variations. Outside London, the available evidence suggests that there are not significant differences, between regions, in the cost of obtaining manpower and there appears to be no available information about possible geographical variations in the cost of obtaining goods and services.

The third and final major defect of the RAWP approach concerns the implicit assumption that equal allocations implies equal provision of health services. This ignores possible variations in the efficiency with which health authorities utilise resources and consequently it is possible that two health authorities with identical resources provide different levels of service, as a result of different levels of efficiency. It has been suggested that variations in the bed occupancy of hospitals are a partial indicator of efficiency and that the RAWP target of a health authority should be reduced it it failed to achieve a pre-determined target of efficiency. While this idea may be worth pursuing, it would seem a difficult task to devise adequate measures of efficiency that would be acceptable to all concerned. Bed occupancy itself is not reliable because of its dependence on factors other than efficiency. For example, a health authority might show a low bed occupancy as a result of its inability to recruit the specialist staff needed to admit and discharge patients as quickly as desired.

3.8 Medical and Dental Teaching Costs and Super-Regional Specialities

Although the factors discussed previously are the main ones in resource allocation within the NHS, we need to mention two additional factors, namely the service increment for teaching (SIFT) which reflects the cost of medical and dental teaching and secondly the method of financing super-regional specialities. The NHS has a statutory responsibility to provide clinical facilities in teaching hospitals, for the teaching of medical and dental students. The direct costs of their education within the medical schools will be funded by the University Grants Committee but the NHS must provide teaching facilities within the hospitals. It is generally accepted that teaching hospitals cost more to run than equivalent non-teaching hospitals and that the additional costs result from the need to provide these teaching facilities. Since the provision of medical education benefits the country as a whole and not just one particular RHA, it seems equitable that a sum of money should be provided to the authorities involved, in order to cover these excess costs of providing teaching facilities. This sum, known as the SIFT, is excluded from the RAWP process and thus protected from redistribution.

The approach taken by the RAWP was to establish the additional cost burden on authorities for each medical or dental student. The cost burden for medical students was assessed by comparing the estimated cost of teaching hospitals with the standard costs of similar non-teaching hospitals as calculated using the '45 Sample Hospital Formula'. The costs for 1977/78 are shown in Table 4.

Table 4 – Excess Cost Burden Per Medical Student in Teaching Hospitals

All figures at 1979-80 prices

Medical School	Estimated relevant costs 1977-78 £'000 (1)	Baseline service costs £'000 (2)	Excess costs (1)-(2) £'000 (3)	Clinical medical students 1979-80 numbers (4)	Excess cost per student £'000 (5)
Westminster	23,097	17,237	5,860	189	31.0
St. Thomas'	18,785	13,425	5,360	213	25.2
Royal Free	16,837	11,169	5,668	242	23.4
St George's	21,104	15,731	5,373	231	23.3
Guy's	17,874	12,146	5,728	255	22.5
Oxford	18,572	15,255	3,317	168	19.7
St Mary's	17,011	12,739	4,272	229	18.7
Cambridge	13,324	11,058	2,266	123	18.4
University College	21,263	16,955	4,308	236	18.3
St Bartholomew's	25,111	18,896	6,215	353	17.6
Charing Cross	14,684	9,532	5,152	315	16.4
London	18,438	13,913	4,525	301	15.0
Median					14.9
King's College	18,763	15,034	3,729	253	14.7
Middlesex	21,917	17,928	3,989	271	14.7
Bristol	32,787	27,812	4,975	348	14.3
Southampton	17,345	13,694	3,651	255	14.3
Manchester	54,188	47,646	6,542	520	12.6
Birmingham	47,653	43,441	4,212	394	10.7
Liverpool	45,370	41,182	4,188	405	10.3
Nottingham	21,893	19,542	2,351	244	9,6
Newcastle	25,322	23,066	2,256	273	8.3
Sheffield	38,862	37,073	1,789	330	5.4
Leicester	22,678	21,816	862	174	4.9
Leeds	27,609	26,865	744	344	2.2
Totals/Average	600,487	503,155	97,332	6,666	14.6

For dental students the excess cost is calculated separately on the basis that 85% of the out-patient costs of dental teaching hospitals is attributed to teaching.

It will be noted that the excess cost burden per student varies greatly between hospitals. It is argued, however, that the excess cost burden is not wholly attributable to the need to provide teaching facilities. Other reasons postulated for this excess are:

(a) the location of regional specialities in teaching hospitals;
(b) research work concentrated in teaching hospitals; and
(c) the tendency for teaching hospitals to be centres of clinical excellence.

Because of the possible effect of these other factors on the running costs of teaching hospitals, the RAWP recommendations were based on compromise and decided to use the median cost per student as the basis for calculating the excess costs of teaching.

Since SIFT only concerns itself with the excess costs of teaching, it is necessary to dis-aggregate the median excess cost per student into the teaching element and the non-teaching element. Due to the lack of information about the excess cost of teaching, the RAWP had to rely on a York University study which suggested that 75% of the excess costs of teaching hospitals can be attributed to the teaching function. The calculation of a national sum for SIFT can therefore be summarised as:

SIFT=Medium excess cost per student $\times$ 75% $\times$ projected number of students.

Minor adjustments to this national SIFT figure are then made to reflect the London weighting and market forces. This national SIFT is then distributed amongst RHAs in proportion to the teaching activity undertaken.

There has been much controversy about the correctness of the SIFT method of funding and we discuss here some of the points made:

(a) It is contended that the York University study has underestimated the proportion of the excess costs of teaching hospitals that is attributable to the teaching functions. A recent report concluded, however, that in the absence of any additional information there was no alternative but to continue to use the 75% figure. Clearly further research on this aspect of teaching hospital costs is desirable.
(b) The basis of the calculation of the excess costs of teaching was reviewed by the Advisory Group on Resource Allocation (AGRA) using 1977/78 data. This also reflected an increase in the number of hospitals where clinical teaching is undertaken and it was recommended that these developments be taken into account when calculating the excess cost of teaching hospitals.

(c) It is suggested that statistics on the excess costs of teaching hospitals do not always reflect the additional burdens on those hospitals resulting from the provision of clinical teaching. However, this is only opinion and we know of no evidence to confirm or deny this suggestion.

Turning now to super-regional specialties, it may be useful to start by defining the term. These specialties are services which are not economically viable nor clinically effective unless they are provided for a population which is substantially larger than that of any one region. The provision of such services by one DHA will obviously distort its financial position when priorities for super-regional specialties have to be matched against the priorities for local services.

Following a recommendation from AGRA, from 1980-81 up to and including 1983-84 adjustments were made to RAWP targets for RHAs providing designated regional specialties in recognition of the additional costs involved. However these arrangements were considered unsatisfactory as they affected only target allocations and in 1983 the Super-Regional Services Advisory Group (SRSAG) was established to advise the Secretary of State on the identification of services to be funded super-regionally and on the appropriate level of provision. The new financing arrangements agreed involved excluding the cost of the four designed super-regional specialties from the RAWP calculation and hence protecting it from redistribution through the RAWP process. As for SIFT the sum protected was added back to RHAs allocations as part of the make up of the cash limit. The SRSAG will continue to advise the Secretary of State on super-regional services. The four specialties currently designated and protected are paediatric haemodialysis and transplantations; spinal injuries services; services for the management of chorion carcinoma and the national poisons information service. The Group has also identified infant and neonatal cardiac surgery as a super-regional service but funds for this service will not be protected through the RAWP system in 1984-85.

3.9   Applying the RAWP Approach

The then Secretary of State adopted the RAWP approach to resource allocation, but also established the AGRA. This group had the task of improving the RAWP methodology within the RAWP principles. Many of the AGRA recommendations have been implemented, such as the adjustment for differences in labour costs between regions. We can therefore say that the DHSS calculates RHA revenue targets by means of a modified RAWP approach. It must be noted, however that the AGRA was disbanded before its work was completed.

Calculation of RHA target allocations is however only one side of the story. When the DHSS has compiled the revenue targets of the RHAs, it can begin the process of distributing the revenue. It begins with the total planned revenue spending for health authorities included in the public expenditure white paper, as adjusted for any last minute changes expressed in the Parliamentary Estimates. This total planned spending is divided into two main parts. First, an amount is set aside for the start figures of each RHA and earmarked allocations such as SIFT, super-regional services and joint finance. These are updated for pay and price increases.

These start figures are used as the base for any general reductions, such as those for efficiency savings, producing a starting point on which a percentage growth addition is applied when any additional revenue is distributed. This growth money is also considered in two parts. Growth in the earmarked allocations is set to one side, and again a balance remains.

Such divisions of the development addition are not mechanistic, but reflect some of the priorities of the Secretary of State. For example, the considerable expansion of the amounts set aside for joint finance over recent years reflects the Secretary of State's emphasis on the value of such spending.

RHA development additions are arrived at by reference to the RAWP target league table. The RHAs which are over target usually receive small increases; those which are under target usually receive large increases. For example, in 1983/84 the most under target RHA, East Anglian received 1.9% growth, while at the other extreme, North West Thames RHA, suffered a reduction of 0.7%. For comparison the national growth rate was 0.21%

To arrive at the final RHA allocations the amount for SIFT and super-regional services is added back. Subsequently, amounts for the earmarked allocations such as joint finance are added.

To conclude our discussion of the RAWP approach to resource allocation let us consider to what extent it fulfills the criteria of a good system of resource allocation, as outlined at the start of this chapter. Firstly equity: it appears to us that since the RAWP approach is concerned, primarily, with the identification, and ultimately the eradication, of inequality in resources between RHA's it broadly fulfills the criterion of equity. Secondly, objectivity: we believe that the RAWP approach is an objective method of resource allocation. Although it is possible to disagree with the composition of the RAWP formula, given a particular formula, there can be little dispute about the size of each target. Thirdly, simplicity: the RAWP approach can not be regarded as simple. We should imagine that there are relatively few people in the country who fully understand the intricacies of the formula and consequently it would be difficult to explain the method to the average member of the public.

3.10 Alternatives to the RAWP Approach

While we broadly favour the RAWP approach, there remains a substantial body of opinion that would prefer an alternative approach. Those against RAWP have often alleged that it lacks flexibility and that it is used too mechanically. Consequently they see it as unable to provide a level of resources consistent with a particular planned or existing level of service. In this section we consider three alternative approaches.

In judging these alternatives we have measured them against the three general principles of resource allocations set out at the beginning of this chapter, namely equity, objectivity and simplicity.

The first of these is an improved statistical model that reflects the need for resources. This is similar in principle to the RAWP approach in that it is concerned with the geographic inequality of resource distribution. The other two assume totally different criteria. One, the use of the NHS Planning System, disregards regional deprivation and allocates resources by taking account of the distribution between client groups. The other method specifically finances approved developments and adopts the principle of providing adequate resources to meet agreed levels of service.

3.11 Improved Needs Model

We have noted that the RAWP approach to resource allocation identified the relative need for resources to provide health services in each region, and that this became the basis for allocating to RHA's the resources available. This RAWP approach has been criticised on many grounds but mainly in relation to the validity of the formula as a measure of relative need. While it is possible to generate improvements to the formula on the basis of improved input data, this would still retain the basis of the RAWP approach and so would not deal with the criticism. We therefore ask whether it would not be possible to base RHA allocations on measures of relative need but to improve the method of calculation by using a completely different approach, namely by using the data base of the RHA strategic plans.

It has been pointed out that the starting point for any corporate plan must be the measurement of the community's need for services. A similar agrument applies to RHA strategic plans: the starting point is, or should be, the process of ascertaining the needs of the community for health services. This is necessarily a rather elaborate process and involves the collection of large volumes of statistical data about the community served. For example, we suggest the following might be included as indicators of the need for health services and could be reflected in an improved needs model, in addition to factors used by the RAWP:

(a) social structure of population
(b) unemployment
(c) other measures of morbidity such as waiting lists
(d) housing standards
(e) population density
(f) industrial pollution.

Once information about these measures of need have been collected, it might then be possible to utilise them for resource allocation purposes. One approach might be to construct a mathematical model which would combine all the various parameters into an overall measure of need, but this becomes really nothing more than a sort of super-RAWP approach. One also has the problem of deciding which of the various need factors is the most important and how they should be weighted. Another approach might be for the DHSS to extract the various measures of need from the RHAs strategic plans and then make explicit subjective decisions as to which RHAs have the relatively greatest need for additional resources. Allocations could be made accordingly.

It could be argued that this method of resource allocation provides for greater equity than the RAWP approach. More sophisticated and appropriate measures of need are used and consequently the overall need of the RHA would be more accurately reflected than by the RAWP approach. Nevertheless, in our opinion, it would prove to be a completely impractical approach due to the inherent lack of objectivity. Ultimately, the decisions about the overall need would be a subjective one and while this might prove to be less rigid than the RAWP approach, the final result would seldom be universally acceptable. Finally, it can be rejected on the grounds of simplicity, in that the procedures involved would be more difficult to grasp than those of the RAWP approach. In addition we see the collection and processing of data as being a very time-consuming process.

3.12 Using the NHS Planning System

The previous two methods of resource allocation have both been concerned with the assessment of need by using statistical data as the basis for distributing resources between RHAs. The essence of this process has been the attempt to eradicate regional inequalities in resource availability. This, however, is not the only possible approach to resource allocation.

A completely different approach to resource allocations could be used, which pays much less attention to these regional inequalities and concentrates on distributing resources between RHAs according to their degree of conformity with national policies and priorities, as expressed through the NHS Planning System.

Using the NHS Planning System to allocate resources essentially implies that revenue will be made available to RHAs as an acknowledgement that the regional priorities and plans conform to the Secretary of State's national strategy and should therefore be supported financially. For example, if a RHA submitted a regional strategy which included the provision of a number of new community units for the mentally handicapped, then over an appropriate period, the Secretary of State would allocate a development addition to the RHA, so that additional finance would be available for the proposal. The development addition would not necessarily be earmarked to the projects, nor would the amount of the development addition be derived from the additional cost of the proposal. It would be in recognition that the projects have the general financial support of the Secretary of State. An example of the other extreme would be a RHA that submits a regional strategy which does not conform to the Secretary of State's preferences. In these circumstances, the RHA would receive no development addition. This would ensure that the health services in their region do not develop in a direction that conflicts with the national view of priorities.

This process is similar to some of the methods used elsewhere in the public sector. In particular, the Department of the Environment allocates resources annually by referring to local priority statements expressed in County Councils' Transport Policies and Programmes, and in the District Councils' Housing Investment Programmes. To decide if such an approach should be used to allocate revenue to RHAs, it is important to establish if such a system would work in the NHS, and if it can, *is it an improvement on the RAWP approach?*

To implement this alternative, the NHS Planning System would require considerable development in respect of the financial information required by the DHSS. We envisage that the most important element for resource allocation purposes would be a detailed revenue programme for, say, the forthcoming five years. This would reveal how the existing revenue monies are being, and will be, spent between client groups in the region. It would also show how anticipated development additions would be used, and spending reductions achieved, again analysing by client groups and including revenue required for new capital schemes. Two points emerge from this requirement. One is that the RHA will have to rearrange the conventional accounting structure of the NHS, and convert this into an analysis similar to that required by a programme budgeting (PB) system. As we show in Chapter 7, this would produce an analysis of spending by client groups. The precise nature and structure of the analysis would obviously have to conform with that required by the DHSS.

Secondly, RHAs would have to submit spending programmes within resource assumptions. This requirement lays a responsibility on the Secretary of State to express a firm view of future growth in NHS resources. A five year forecast would be needed in order to relate revenue requirements to the capital programme. After reading about the PESC methodology in Chapter 2 this may seem to be a relatively easy task, but such forecasts of growth for regions over the forthcoming years have not always been readily available. This lack of information would have to be rectified, and forecasts produced, however tenuous. Otherwise the RHAs submissions, when aggregated, could be so unrealistic as to make the exercise valueless.

How would the RHAs programmes be judged? The answer would depend on the aims of the Secretary of State and his priorities. While one eye could be kept on geographic equality the other would be looking for the shift in emphais towards those services considered to be of high priority. This potentially double-edged approach highlights the great advantage of this method; it can be used to achieve a distribution of resources in both geographic and client-group terms. The scope of this financial influence in achieving the implementation of national priorities cannot be overstated. Because the RAWP approach only operates at the geographic level, it is therefore more limited in its potential.

One drawback of the approach is its dependence on bureaucracy. Annually, DHAs would have to provide information to enable the RHA to compile bids for submission to the DHSS. The DHSS could not possibly hope to consider every proposal, so the minor proposals could be grouped, and major proposals, however defined, be readily identified. Such a process can be very susceptible to political influence. Some RHAs are likely to exert greater influence over the approval of proposals. Similarly, the more influential RHAs will be able to exert their will as to the financial support to be given to the approved proposals. For example, imagine the dilemma of the Secretary of State in choosing between two proposals, one to spend on acute services in a deprived RHA, the other to spend on services for the mentally handicapped in a well provided RHA. Dilemmas can easily be exploited by clandestine political influence. In this respect the RAWP approach can stand above the political arena to a much greater degree.

A related difficulty is for those RHAs who may have to deal with development additions which are less than anticipated: a position likely to arise frequently. One way in which they can be consistent with the national process is to rank the DHAs proposals in order of priority and allocate the development addition to DHAs in sequence. As in the national context, within a region, DHAs will have the opportunity to exert their political will and to influence the outcome, the intention being to corner the market in resources. Once again, the influential DHAs are likely to further improve their position, an opportunity not so readily available when using RAWP principles.

If development additions were earmarked to specific proposals, controls would need to be devised to ensure that the money is not diverted to other purposes. A bureaucratic system would have to extend from the DHSS to each RHA, and probably on to each DHA in order to account for the use of any development addition. The NHS has been notoriously bad in this respect. Many earmarked allocations have often been used, either wholly or partly, for purposes beyond the use specified. Before such a process as outlined here could be implemented, a considerable improvement in the financial control of the NHS would be required.

Finally, we come to our three general principles of resource allocation and how this method fits in with them. Firstly, equity: this method ignores regional inequalities in favour of client group inequalities. These cannot yet be measured adequately, so we consider that it fails in this respect. Secondly, the criteria of objectivity is not met by allocation methods such as these. While many of the programmes may be based on an extensive analysis of objective data, an objective comparison between RHAs may not be possible because RHAs may use different data bases. For example, one RHA may wish to proceed with a development based on a demonstrable improvement in access rates, while another may justify a proposal by using workload statistics. The process fails our test of objectivity because it is not possible to agree which objective data is the most appropriate to take into account, or to give, particular emphasis. Furthermore, while such a method, based on priority preferences, can work in the NHS, and may be appropriate in other parts of the public sector, we do not consider that it is appropriate for the allocation process between the DHSS and RHAs. The main advantage is its susceptibility to political influence and opportunism. Such wheeling and dealing operated before the RAWP method was introduced and the limitations can be demonstrated by the currently skewed distribution of resources between RHAs. Finally, as noted earlier, this approach to resource allocation would probably prove to be a bureaucratic nightmare and so can be condemmed on the grounds of lack of simplicity.

3.13 Revenue Consequences of Capital Schemes (RCCS)

The third alternative that we have considered here takes RCCS as its criterion for distributing the development addition. One of the main demands on any extra revenue for the NHS is the cost of opening new capital schemes. In particular, it is generally accepted that even replacing old hospitals with new ones requires more revenue, because the technology of modern hospital buildings is such that they cost more to run than old buildings. A further aspect to take into account is that the most significant expansion of health services, in terms of cost, arises from the provision of new buildings, particularly hospitals. This can be referred to as an expansion of the infrastructure. The justification for this approach to allocating revenue is consistency. Having supported the expansion of the infrastructure, by providing the capital (and in the case of larger hospitals actually approved the scheme in detail) the Secretary of State is not being consistent if he does not subsequently provide an appropriate sum of revenue so that the buildings can be commissioned.

Estimates of RCCS produced by each DHA and aggregated by the RHA would provide the information for the process. This information is already available to RHAs, and could be easily provided to the DHSS. Each RHA would then be given a development addition which corresponds with the RCCS submission.

If any development addition remains unallocated after the RCCS has been financed, it can be distributed between RHAs either by using RAWP principles or by financing specific proposals. If the development addition is insufficient to meet the total RCCS of the RHAs then presumably the amount available would be distributed pro-rata to submissions, leaving each RHA with the problem of financing the shortfall.

This process is extremely simple to understand and operate and this is its main advantage. Each RHA knows what it must do in order to attain an increase in resources, and can easily see why other RHAs have been given more. It therefore passes our test of objectivity.

Problems arise, however, when we come to consider the equity of this approach. The main objection concerns the dependence on the capital allocation process. It seems to be inappropriate that the allocation of part of the revenue of the NHS should depend on the principles used to allocate capital. Any inequalities in the distribution of revenue will not necessarily be corrected by this approach. No mechanism exists to ensure that the more deprived regions will be allocated a greater share of capital and thus be able to attract a greater share of any development addition.

A further objection to this approach is the emphasis given to RCCS as having a prior claim. Some people consider that a more important priority is to provide additional revenue so that the 'cinderella services' can be expanded. Financing RCCS would tend to perpetuate existing inequalities because most major capital schemes would tend to be related to the general and acute services. It may be possible to improve some of the 'cinderella services' by expanding community services, which require little or no capital and would therefore not attract additional resources.

Another problem with this approach is its lack of uniformity in estimating the cost of RCCS. It can be assessed by using the 45 Sample Hospital Formula, so making the basis of RCCS figures of each RHA comparable. Whether the norms are appropriate to each capital scheme is debatable. Usually norms, by their nature, are not directly applicable in specific situations and consequently RCCS estimates based on these might not prove sufficiently accurate. Even more significant are the financial effects of any savings arising from new capital schemes as such savings must be deducted from the RCCS estimate before submission is made. Unfortunately, no standard method exists for the calculation of such savings and so RHAs can choose from a number of methods. It is obviously in the interests of the RHA to minimise any savings, and the choice of the costing method may well reflect this factor.

The vagaries of RCCS calculations make them unreliable as a means of allocating development additions to RHAs. Their use would be unlikely to result in more fair distributions of revenue, but would only resolve the Treasurers problems of financing his health authority's RCCS. We see no merit in this approach.

These alternatives are considered in Chapter 6 in the context of allocating revenue from RHAs to DHAs. At this level their use has different implications. Our general dismissal of their use nationally in favour of the RAWP approach should not be taken as an indication of a complete dismissal of their use within RHAs.

3.14   Capital Allocations to RHAs

Capital allocations are intended to finance the capital expenditure of health authorities. While capital expenditure has a precise accounting definition, it will suffice here to point out that, broadly, it is spending on items such as land, buildings, and expensive items of equipment.

While this broad description of capital expenditure conforms, generally, to that in other organisations, capital allocations to RHAs have an important peculiarity: the capital monies used by RHAs are free of interest and do not have to be repaid. It is not a loan, but an allocation synonymous with a grant which can be used to finance capital expenditure. The monies are handed over by the DHSS to the health authorities during the financial year, the health authorities having no power to borrow through capital money markets.

Four main methods of allocating capital are considered here. They are:
(a) the method preferred by the RAWP
(b) the way the RAWP proposals are being implemented by the DHSS
(c) the bidding approach considered by the RAWP
(d) a brief outline of a NHS Planning System approach.

3.15   The RAWP Method – Capital Stock

The capital allocation process recommended by the RAWP follows similar principles to those used in its revenue approach. It uses targets to express the need for capital facilities and compares this with the existing facilities in order to highlight any relative deprivation. The first step in the process is to value each RHAs capital stock.

Capital stock could have been valued with great precision, such as a comprehensive review and valuation of existing land, buildings and equipment, rather like a stock take. However, the RAWP rejected such an approach in preference to a simple rule of thumb. For example, hospitals in existence at the end of 1961 were valued by using an estimated replacement cost for each bed. This, of course, does not just mean the replacement cost of the actual beds themselves, but reflects the value of the whole hospital in which the beds are located. To this was added the actual capital expenditure since 1961. The resulting amount was depreciated to reflect the wear and tear on these assets. The valuation excludes assets such as ambulance stations and land. RAWP considered that these omitted items were broadly distributed in the same proportion as hospital beds, and that such an assumption would not seriously distort the accuracy of the resulting capital stock value.

The second step in the capital RAWP process is to calculate a notional stock target for each RHA. This is calculated, by distributing the value of the total NHS capital stock, pro-rata to an appropriate RAWP weighted population for each RHA. When the stock target is compared with the actual stock value, the over- and under-target position is revealed. The process is illustrated in Table 5 using two hypothetical RHAs.

Comparison of the RHAs actual capital stock with its notional stock target will show to what degree the RHA is above or below its capital RAWP target. It is important to realise that these stock figures should not be

Table 5 — Calculation of Target Stock

RHA	Actual Stock £ million	Weighted population million	Target Stock £ million	Over/under target £ million
A	250	4	200	+50 over-target
B	250	6	300	- 50 under-target
	500	10	500	

confused with the actual allocation of capital monies received each year by the RHA. Clearly the capital allocation, and hence the capital expenditure, will increase the size of the RHAs capital stock and consequently capital allocations to RHAs can be set in such a way as to raise under-target RHAs to their RAWP target. Where the amount of the national capital allocation is small, the move towards targets will also be small.

Progress towards these targets was considered by the RAWP, which suggested that any redistribution of resources be completed as quickly as possible. It recommended three matters to be borne in mind:

(a) each RHAs capacity to absorb extra capital
(b) the need to ensure that over-target RHAs have a capital allocation which is large enough to permit it to meet its commitments, while having an adequate amount of uncommitted capital to replenish old capital stock
(c) the need for a smooth transition.

One factor not recognised by the RAWP is the rigidity of capital. While the distribution of capital allocations can be varied at will, infrastructure cannot be switched between the RHAs; it cannot be uprooted and moved. One clear example is the supposedly excess teaching hospital in London. Even if it were possible to close one of the teaching hospitals, it is not possible to move it physically to another part of the country.

The approach outlined by the RAWP for implementing its proposals was to use a set minimum level of capital which could be allocated to each RHA without regard to any relative shortfall. This would cover any contractual commitments and planned spending. For the two years following the RAWP report, 1977/78 and 1978/79, the recommended set minimum was 90% and 80% respectively of the available capital funds. After these years a progressively larger proportion would be allocated using the RAWP formula, so that eventually 90% of the available capital would be allocated on a weighted population basis. A ceiling was suggested to ensure that no RHA received an allocation that was too large to spend sensibly. This was to be related to the share, of total capital available, that each RHA could expect to receive if all the capital were distributed in proportion to the weighted population. For the first year, 1977/78, a ceiling of 110% of the population-based share was recommended, rising in annual steps of 10% up to a maximum ceiling of 140%.

3.16   Capital RAWP – Weighted Populations

As we have already mentioned, capital targets are derived from a distribution of the NHS capital stock between RHAs by using a weighted population. There are four main differences between the weighted population used for calculating capital targets and that used for calculating revenue targets. They are in respect of the population base; cross boundary flows; community services; and FPC administration.

The population base is designed to reflect the need to provide infra-structure for a future population and RAWP preferred to use the population which was expected five years hence. It considered that such a projection would balance the requirement to provide infrastructure for a future population with the inherent risk of error and uncertainty in longer term projections. Similarly, the RAWP believed that the weightings in the revenue formula of age/sex utilisation and mortality patterns could be applied to a five-year projection without significant distortion.

As we mentioned previously, cross-boundary flows were used in the RAWP's revenue formula. For capital targets, it considered that most inter-regional cross-boundary flows should be disregarded. Exceptions specified by the RAWP included the flows associated with centres of excellence and regional specialties. Such an adjustment infers that in the longer term cross-boundary flows between regions are not desirable, but some, which are outside the scope of the exceptions, may represent sensible management. Examples would be those RHAs which border Wales or Scotland where many sections of the population may sensibly and conveniently turn to English RHAs for services. Similarly, the juxtaposition of towns and communities with neighbouring RHAs may make the flows a desirable and permanent feature of access to health services.

In the revenue target the weighted population for community services uses an age weighting of the actual population to reflect the use of health services rather than infrastructure. For the capital targets the RAWP recommended an age weighting of GP consultation. While RAWP acknowledged that this weighting may not be fully comprehensive it considered that it would represent a better measure of the uptake of the community services infrastructure.

FPC administration excludes items such as GPs and dentists surgeries and consequently consumes a minimal amount of capital. The RAWP suggested that this element could be omitted from the formula, leaving six separate weighted populations which are combined into a single weighted population for each RHA. The combination of these weighted populations also differs from the revenue target. It is based on the estimated national proportions of capital spending of each of the six service aspects for the following three years. The total value of NHS capital is then distributed in proportion to this combined weighted population to give a stock target for each RHA.

3.17   Actual Capital Allocations

Having described the RAWP suggestion for capital allocations, we turn to the actual approach currently used at the DHSS. As with most broad principles, when they are applied, some refinement is required. So it is with the RAWPs approach to capital; the DHSS have adopted the principles but with modifications in the way they have been applied.

The aims of the allocation process used by the DHSS are initially to achieve approximate equity between RHAs and thereafter to continue to make future allocations which will maintain the balance between each region's capital stock relative to its need for capital. The DHSS has reviewed the progress made in achieving these aims and have been able to refine the allocation process. Some of the issues considered are outlined here.

As regards the formula itself, the RAWP method of weighting the population of each RHA has been adopted with only minor changes by the DHSS, such as, omitting the annual steps of 10% and the smoothing factor increased from 10% to 20%. Three major changes to the stock valuation methodology have been considered. Firstly, adjusting the pre 1962 stock for any permanent reductions in beds in hospitals built before this time. Secondly, this pre 1962 valuation is written down by 10% per annum on a straight-line basis.

Similarly, the effect of capital stock introduced after 1962 should be depreciated more than previously. The depreciation rate suggested by RAWP of 2.5% is seen by the DHSS as too low and a rate of 4% may be more appropriate. Thirdly, the addition to each RHAs capital stock since 1979/80 should be derived from the actual capital allocation made instead of the actual capital expenditure incurred. This would remove the effect of transfers from capital and revenue which can reduce the capital allocated and enable RHAs to distort the attainment of approximate equality. As greater equality in capital between RHA's has been achieved the DHSS now propose that instead of allocating the basic minimum of 85% of the capital in relation to weighted population and 15% using the stock equalisation, the basic minimum should be increased by phasing out the stock equalisation element over 7 years from 1985/86. Thus from 1991/92 and onwards weighted population alone will be the criterion.

One variation is proposed in the calculation which will make the formula more responsive to population change. Regions whose populations are growing at a rate faster than the national average will be given a favourable weighting. This is expected to be an addition to the weighted population of ten times the region's annual growth in population. This adjustment is designed to recognise that population growth results in a proportionately higher need for capital. Finally it is proposed that when the basic minimum allocations are increased above 85%, the level for the four Thames RHAs should be reduced by 2½ points to reflect the capital made available separately to the post-graduate teaching hospitals in London.

This adjustment brings us to the specific capital allocations. These take up about 20% of the total capital available, leaving 80% for general use by RHAs, and can be summarised as follows:

(a) Central Services: this allocation is to finance capital spending at units providing a national service, particularly in the research field. An example is the health service element of Porton Down.

(b) Boards of Governors of University Medical Schools: the agreed capital budgets of the Boards of Governors are financed by an earmarked allocation.

(c) Teaching hospitals: the NHS contributes 35% of the cost of approved teaching hospital schemes, and this is financed from this earmarked allocation. This allocation is therefore associated with the allocation for the boards of Governors.

(d) Dental hospital re-equipment: a fixed allocation is made to each of the ten RHAs which have dental hospitals within their boundaries.

(e) Special schemes: where a health authority proceeds with a capital scheme which may provide a national service, or is of research interest, or is a national priority, may be financed from this allocation.

(f) Inner cities: those RHAs within which inner city partnerships or programme arrangements have been established receive an allocation from this pool. It is based on the amount previously identified as the minimum spending on primary care services.

(g) Urban Programme: partnership and programme authorities are also involved in implementing the Urban Programme. An allocation is made from this pool on the basis of bids approved by the Department of the Environment.

(h) Strategic shift: this represents an interest free loan to finance capital spending identified in a RHAs strategic plan, but which exceeds the capital allocation available for the year. Such loans are repaid from the RHAs future capital allocation, and the amount repaid reflects inflation over the period. While interest is not charged, the addition for inflation means that the loan repayments are similar to those for conventional borrowing arrangements.

(i) Over- and under-spending: these are carried forward to the next financial year. In addition joint finance for capital purposes is added and any adjustments made for brokerage. This is where an RHA may wish to give up some of its capital until a future year and the amount is loaned to another RHA. The DHSS may use a broking pool which may involve several RHAs.

3.18   The Bidding Approach

The RAWP considered one alternative to the capital targets approach and this was the bidding approach. It reflected the extent to which health authorities were prepared to sacrifice revenue in order to pay for capital and therefore has, as its major advantage, an approximation to a capital money market that is experienced by other organisations in the private and public sector. The revenue sacrifice is a proxy for the interest rate paid by these other agencies, and so the bidding approach is designed to improve the utilisation of capital, which at present is free to health authorities.

Not a great deal of detail about the mechanics of the bidding approach was included in the RAWP report. In outline, the system would seem to work by RHAs, presumably after consultation with DHAs, ranking capital schemes in priority groups such as very urgent; urgent; less urgent, each of which has an annual notional rate of return for 20 years, of say 12%: 10%: 8% respectively. If a RHA wishes to pursue a very urgent scheme, it would therefore be prepared to sacrifice 12% of the capital cost from each of its revenue allocations for the next 20 years. The total capital available would be distributed by allocating sufficient capital to finance the very urgent schemes. Any balance remaining would then be used to finance the urgent schemes and so on until all the capital was used. RHAs with successful bids would suffer the agreed reduction in revenue.

The great merit of this proposal is its links with the revenue allocation process. The RAWP envisaged that the revenue repaid to the DHSS could be available to redistribute to the RHAs using the RAWP revenue allocation formula. A much quicker redistribution of revenue resources was envisaged if the bidding approach was used instead of the capital targets approach, because revenue monies amounting to some 10% of the capital allocation would be available to increase the development addition.

Other advantages of the bidding approach are first: it allows RHAs to determine their own ratios of capital to revenue resources. They can choose to receive a large capital allocation at the expense of revenue, or keep their revenue allocations high but have a small capital allocation. Consequently central decisions about the relative requirements of health authorities are not required. Second: because of the link between capital and revenue resources, RHAs are encouraged to appraise all capital investment decisions in terms of well established techniques such as discounted cash flow (DCF). In fact such appraisals may be more meaningful than when capital is free to health authorities. Third: within the limits of the process, RHAs can to some extent determine their own pace of movement towards equality. For example, under-capitalised RHAs can choose to improve their infrastructure by foregoing revenue. Conversely, a RHA that is deprived of revenue can choose to forego capital and so minimise its interest repayments, and increase the revenue available to improve levels of service.

The major disadvantage of the method is its bureaucratic complexity. A great deal of detailed information has to be collected not just from RHAs but from DHAs beforehand, and this may prove too cumbersome to be effective. Furthermore, the annual capital auction casts a large degree of uncertainty on future capital schemes as they emerge from spending programmes and queue up for finance in the current year. The RAWP recognised that this method may be more workable and appropriate for allocating capital from RHAs to DHAs, and it seems to us that this is probably its most appropriate role.

3.19   Using the NHS Planning System

Another alternative to the RAWP targets method could be referred to as the NHS Planning System approach. As we outlined previously for revenue allocations, appropriate acceptable capital spending programmes would provide the basis, and capital would be allocated to finance those schemes that conform to national priorities. If a RHA submitted proposals which did not conform to national priorities, the capital required would not be allocated to that RHA by the DHSS. A little more is said about this approach in Chapter 6 in relation to capital allocations to DHAs, but the principles at either regional or district level are similar.

For expediency, the first requirement would probably be to allocate capital directly to large schemes, then to allocate a block of capital for smaller unidentified schemes. This will reduce the number of schemes to be considered individually by the DHSS. Clearly, multi-million pound schemes should be considered by the DHSS. However, below such a value the distinction is much less clear. For example, some schemes of say £1 million may be critical in implementing national priorities. The DHSS would have to decide how far it wished to exercise direct influence over the future of individual schemes. Currently, schemes costing more than £5 million are reviewed by the DHSS in respect of matters such as design and content. It may be convenient to use a similar dividing line.

One aspect to consider with this alternative is the method by which the DHSS will divide the capital available between larger schemes and smaller schemes. No magical formula can be suggested to help in this decision and the main principles would tend to be similar to those outlined in Chapter 2. The personal preference of the Secretary of State or the Governments policies would determine the emphasis. An influencing factor could be the amount of revenue available to the NHS which may limit the new developments which can be afforded. In addition, advances in building technology, particularly in respect of energy conservation, may require replacement rather than developments, which in itself may still require large scale multi-million pound schemes. Whichever factors are operating in any one year, they are likely to change over time, and any allocation process should be responsive to such changes. This requirement almost inevitably leads to a subjective view as to the appropriate split.

By allocating capital specifically to schemes, the DHSS would probably wish to safisfy itself that the capital had been used as envisaged. A system of monitoring would be required with this approach to ensure that RHAs were directly accountable to the DHSS for the use of the capital. This system could prove to be quite cumbersome, as no similar mechanism exists at present, and additional paperwork would be required: a clear disadvantage of this approach.

The distribution of the capital for smaller schemes, in our example costing less than £5 million, presents much more difficulty than the approach for larger schemes. Because the allocation is not specifically linked to schemes or programmes, criteria for distribution are required. For example the RAWP suggested that its revenue weighted population may provide appropriate proportions for distributing such capital, but in our opinion, this measure may not adequately reflect the need for such capital, especially when the costs relating to fairly large capital schemes, could be considerable. An alternative would be to use the RAWPs capital allocation formula.

Clearly, the NHS Planning System cannot by itself provide an adequate means of allocating capital monies to RHAs. An attempt in this direction would result in a considerable amount of bureaucracy and would be cumbersome to operate.

3.20 Earmarked Allocations

About 2% of the resources for health authorities are allocated to RHAs in a different manner to that outlined previously. One difference is that the use of such allocations is specified by the Secretary of State, and a second is that the methods of allocation are often not derived from the RAWP formula. To complete the outline of the allocations to RHAs, we have briefly described two earmarked allocations, joint finance and special development projects:

(a) In 1976 the Secretary of State introduced the joint finance allocation. The intention is to earmark part of the resources for the NHS for the express purpose of financing expansions in the levels of service provided by social service, education and housing authorities, voluntary bodies and community services provided by DHAs. Two particular objectives must be borne in mind in releasing joint finance monies. Firstly, proposals must benefit the NHS by helping to keep people out of hospital. Secondly, projects which transfer people from hospital care into the community can be financed from joint finance monies. This is the 'care in the community' initiative. Such schemes can also be financed from DHAs ordinary revenue cash limit.

The emphasis on the particular types of service gives the basis of the allocation to RHAs. A small proportion of the national allocation is allocated by taking account of the special problems of inner cities. For the balance, equal account is taken of the population over 75 and the use made of hospital facilities for mentally ill and mentally handi-capped patients by the actual age/sex groups.

Initially, the DHSS divides the joint finance allocation between capital and revenue in proportion to the previous year's spending. The eventual actual split is determined by the types of schemes adopted by each DHA. This is considered in Chapter 6.

(b) The second earmarked allocation that we have outlined is for develop-ment projects. These are mainly related to testing the effects of a different method of providing a service. An example, would be the linking of services for the mentally ill and the services for the elderly, perhaps with greater emphasis on the community care provision. Such a change from more conventional institutional care may require a pilot scheme in order to assess and understand the effects of the changes. The revenue costs of such a project could be financed by a specific revenue allocation and this method is used in a small number of cases.

The main purposes of these variations from the RAWP approach is one of aims. Often, the Secretary of State will have a particular policy or innovation he wishes to pursue, and he effectively 'top slices' part of the revenue for the NHS and earmarks this for his purpose. The cash is allocated directly to where he intends it to be used. These earmarked allocations are tending to grow in importance, particularly that for joint finance. It is difficult to envisage an allocation system in which the Secretary of State will not intervene, as it is one of his main tools for shaping and changing services provided to patients.

Most of the allocation methods outlined in this chapter are relevant to the allocation process between RHAs and DHAs. Some are more appropriate at that level and they are considered in this context in Chapter 6.

3.21 The Allocation Process in Scotland and Wales

One major distinction between England and both Scotland and Wales can be attributed to the difference in structures. In Scotland and Wales the lack of RHAs results in allocations being made directly to the operational tier of the health authority or board. While the formulae used have been based on the RAWP principles they have been modified to take account of this structural difference. The modification process can be seen as similar to the changes implemented by RHAs before using the RAWP formula to allocate revenue to DHAs, although in Wales the formula has been used purely as an indicator of inequality of provision which then attracts additional resources, rather than as a basis for the redistribution of resources.

Taking revenue first, the Scottish approach is based on the Scottish Health Authorities Revenue Equalisation (SHARE) report. In Wales, the formula is based on the work of the Steering Committee on Resource Allocations in Wales (SCRAW) which has been replaced by the Working Group on Resource Allocation. This has a wider remit covering matters relevant to the allocation of NHS resources in Wales. One element of its role is to monitor the formula for assessing the relative financial position between DHAs developed by SCRAW, as the Secretary of State for Wales has announced his intention of using this formula as the basis for his programme of eliminating inequalities in DHA resources by 1985/86. Towards this end he has made available significant sums of additional resources.

The SHARE formula combines six populations, namely non-psychiatric in-patients; obstetric in-patients (which are combined in the RAWP formula); mental illness in-patients; mental subnormality in-patients; day and out-patients and community health services. The ambulance service and FPC admininstration populations used in the RAWP formula are not included in the SHARE formula.

Four interesting differences from the RAWP approach are worthy of note. Firstly, a sparsity factor is used for community health services by using nurses travelling time proportion and information from the Scottish Rural Practices Fund. Secondly, special allowance is made for pre 1969 long stay mentally ill and mentally sub-normal patients.

Thirdly, an adjustment is made to reflect the additional cost burdens borne by those equivalent DHAs which have super district beds. In these respects, the formula recognises some of the more precise effects of allocating revenue directly to the operational tier of the NHS rather than to RHAs.

Perhaps the most substantial difference between RAWP and SHARE is in the use of SMRs. SHARE rejected the RAWP method of using separate SMRs for each of the 17 disease classifications and preferred the all-causes SMR for each age group. This is intended to neutralise the effect of small changes in total deaths producing large savings in weighted populations. For example 20% of total mortality was attributed to almost half the beds in Scotland and changes in th 20% could therefore have a marked affect on the formula.

The SCRAW approach differs from the RAWP formula in one major element. The SCRAW does not recommend the use of a formula to assess the need for psychiatric nor mental handicap services although the exclusion of these services from the formula is currently being reviewed. In addition, the FPC administration element is also not used in Wales. The Welsh view of SMRs does not correspond to the English view as the SCRAW has recommended that crude and not specific condition SMRs are incorporated into the formula. Two further Welsh factors are worthy of note, namely, the sparsity factor for the ambulance element and an adjustment has been made for seasonal population savings attributable to tourism. The four populations used in the SCRAW approach are for in-patients; out-patients; community health and ambulance services.

Omitting the psychiatric element from the formula is matched by special allocations for psychiatric services which reflect the need for finance, and this is a particularly significant matter as the Welsh system combines both a 'needs formula' and a 'planning system' approach to resource allocation.

Significantly, the SHARE and SCRAW say little about the allocation of capital. In Wales, the process has been one of bidding for capital, not on the lines of the RAWP's bidding approach, but essentially requiring each DHA to convince the Welsh Office that their capital schemes were of greater priority than those of their neighbours. From 1984/85, a new method is proposed. Of the total provision for hospital and community health service expenditure in Wales, some 7% will be available for capital. The DHAs share of this will be distributed by using a formula comprised of three elements; an adjusted population element for one quarter of the capital; a replacement factor for one quarter of the capital and an equalisation factor for the remaining half. The aim is to achieve theoretical equality in the distribution of capital assets over 20 years.

In Scotland, capital has been distributed in two ways. About one third of the sum available has been distributed to boards in a manner broadly consistent with the SHARE formula. This has been available for spending on smaller capital schemes. The remaining two thirds has been used to finance the major capital programme which is managed centrally by the Scottish Home and Health Department. At the time of writing the method of allocating capital to boards is being reviewed.

4

Priorities and Planning

4.1 The Distinction between Priorities and Planning

We have already seen in Chapter 2 how the Government attempts to plan the total volume and allocation of public expenditure by using systems such as the PESC procedures. In this chapter we examine the role of the Government, via the DHSS, in determining priorities for health services; and show how it attempts to influence the distribution of resources between the various types of health services. This will involve an examination of the DHSS/NHS interface.

The two terms planning and priorities are often used synonymously. Although they are complementary, they do in fact represent different concepts. It is generally the case that the determination of priorities for the NHS officially falls to the Secretary of State as the policy-maker, while planning is the province of the health authorities, both DHAs and RHAs, Planning is the means by which the Secretary of State's priorities can be translated into RHA and DHA strategies. As this book is not concerned with the Government's policy-making process, we shall not examine, in detail, how priorities for the NHS are formulated We shall, however, consider how effectively those policies are implemented.

Unlike some other parts of the public sector, the NHS has, since 1974, adopted a formal approach to planning. It is referred to as the NHS Planning System and has recently been revised. In this chapter we shall outline the operation and aims of this revised NHS Planning System. In addition we shall examine some of the weaknesses of the NHS Planning System and point out why, in our opinion, it fails to justify its *raison d'etre*. The NHS Planning System rests on the concepts of priorities planning and review. We shall consider each of these in turn.

4.2 Priorities

The Secretary of State is responsible for formulating NHS policy. We see this role as having two main components:

(a) determining policies which are implemented directly by the DHSS; examples include prescription charges, charges for overseas patients, pay beds, DGH size, method of finance
(b) determining policies which are implemented with the co-operation of health authorities; examples are greater emphasis on services for the elderly, mentally ill and mentally handicapped, improved preventive health care, more effective health education. We refer to these kinds of policies as priorities.

Priorities emerge from wider ranging documents such as 'Care in Action'. and are restated in more short term documents such as 'DHSS Planning Guidelines'. This may be interpreted as a 'top down' process, the starting point being the formulation, by the Secretary of State, of a broad policy for the NHS which indicates the overall direction in which the service is intended to develop. To a large extent priorities can be formulated on the basis of information currently available. For example, since current statistics suggest an increasingly high proportion of elderly people in the population, it is essential that priorities reflect the future need to care for these people. Ultimately, however, the NHS is restricted by the resources available to it and consequently choices have to be made.

It is desirable that there should be some rational method for choosing between alternative priorities, and the question is frequently asked: *how, in fact, does the Secretary of State, with the DHSS, select those to be promulgated within the NHS?* Economists may suggest that the methodology for assessing and arriving at a particular priority should be similar to the cost/benefit approach. For each option, the costs and benefits of implementation should be assessed and options ranked in order of greatest net benefit. However, sound information on costs is not always available and estimates may not be sufficiently reliable, so it is not always easy to calculate the costs of various options. The assessment of benefits is infinitely more difficult because of the lack of information on matters such as precisely who benefits, how they benefit, and to what extent. Although considerable research is being undertaken into the provision of such measures at present there is nothing reliable on which to base decisions about priorities. Because of the difficulty in assessing options according to any scientific decision making process, it appears that choices at a national level are heavily influenced by the value

judgements of the relevant Secretary of State. This subjectivity is highlighted by illustrations of unpredictable and unstable priorities which can
often be attributed to political factors such as change in Government. One
main cause is that the politicians responsible for the service, such as the
Secretary of State, are seldom in office for a sufficiently long period to fully
implement their priorities.

An example is the change in policy concerning the size of new hospitals.
For many years, the NHS had been developing services based on large
DGHs, sometimes with more than 1,000 beds, which combined general and
acute services with those for the elderly and the mentally ill. The previous
Government favoured a return to smaller DGHs supported by local hospitals which would include services for acute patients and long-stay
patients. Generally the current Government favours a more centralised
approach.

Although the unpredictability in NHS policy and priorities can cause
problems for the health authorities in planning their services it is a fact of
life which they must tolerate. Governments are democratically elected and
are free to amend policies and priorities irrespective of what previous
Governments have decided. However, it is fair to say that most recent
Governments have been consistent in their policies for increasing
resources available for the 'cinderella services' for the elderly, mentally ill,
mentally handicapped and families.

Clearly, in order that Government priorities for the NHS be implemented, it is necessary that their guidance be incorporated into the plans of
the health authorities. It is essential that guidelines are made available to
health authorities and this is done via documents such as circulars and
DHSS publications. The main document is the annual DHSS Planning
Guidelines. This is issued to RHAs and DHAs, and reflects the national
priorities that should be pursued over the next two years. While it usually
has a two-year perspective, it is seen against the background of a ten-year
strategy. The three main topics dealt with are: capital and revenue assumptions for the forthcoming financial years, manpower assumptions, and the
main national problems to be tackled as perceived by the DHSS.

These national guidelines are open to local interpretation where this may
be thought necessary. Consequently, DHSS Planning Guidelines may be
amended by RHAs and passed to DHAs in the amended form. Unfortunately, there is often a thin line between amending guidelines and replacing them altogether. This will be discussed further in a later section but for
now, we turn to the associated topic of plans.

4.3 Planning

Plan preparation is primarily the responsibility of health authorities. They are required to prepare plans that state their future priorities. Such planning operates simultaneously on two levels. The first is strategy, which culminates in a ten-year strategic plan, to be reviewed every five years by RHAs and DHAs. The health authority's strategy would include its priorities set against resource forecasts for the period. These would be based to varying degrees on planning guidelines.

The second is the operational level, at which planning is more specific and precise. A typical annual programme is prepared by a DHA every year and shows proposed actions for each of the next two years; a plan of action for year one and a programme for year two. However, there are exceptions to this general rule and some health authorities prepare programmes for up to five years in advance, particularly for capital spending.

The links between plans and priorities are clearly that health authorities are required to prepare plans based on local needs and circumstances while at the same time taking note of the relevant priorities expressed in planning guidelines. Logically, of course, it is also necessary that annual programmes are derived from the relevant strategic plan otherwise the whole procedure loses cohesion and structure. DHA plans are reviewed by the RHA and incorporated into the overall strategic plan for the region. RHAs should then submit the strategic plan to the DHSS. In principle, the review is intended only to ensure that these plans generally accord with the planning guidelines. In the light of the regional strategic and operational plans the DHSS will then re-examine its priorities for the future, and if necessary revise its planning guidelines to take account of achievements. A review of planning guidelines does not necessarily mean a change in priorities.

What will happen if a DHA disregards the policy guidelines is not clear. RHAs are required to reconcile DHA's plans, and must hold themselves in readiness to discuss planning matters and priorities as they arise with DHAs. No provision exists for RHAs to direct DHAs to pursue particular priorities, but clearly the RHA can still exert great influence over the priorities of the DHA. For example, the RHA usually controls the capital programme for the region and consequently can decide which schemes are or are not included. Furthermore, it is the RHA who decides the level of DHA revenue funding and it is easy to see how it could exert pressure on a DHA to conform with RHA policy guidelines.

4.4   Performance Review

One major weakness of planning in the NHS was that it did not operate as a cycle. Plans and programmes were prepared and agreed but no-one at a central point took the process further by effectively and regularly reviewing the progress towards implementing the plans and hence producing further information which would feed back into the preparation of subsequent plans. This weakness was corrected in 1982 when the Secretary of State responded to the comments of the Public Accounts Committee.

The arrangements implemented from 1983/84 were for Ministers to lead an annual DHSS review of the plans and programmes of each RHA. In addition, the effectiveness with which resources were used would also be examined. The main aim of the reviews would be to hold RHAs accountable for the implementation of Government policies on matters such as improving the 'cinderalla services' and following the discussions to agree a firm statement on the progress to be achieved in the following year. In this latter respect the reviews clearly produce a feedback for the subsequent annual programme.

A subsequent review process between RHAs and DHAs was also implemented in 1983/84. This followed the same lines as the regional review and essentially completes the process by reconciling national strategic aims for service developments and efficiency with the achievements of management at the operational tier of the DHA. In this respect the review process can be seen as extending from the Secretary of State to each DHA.

It is clear to us that the Public Accounts Committee's criticism of the lack of accountability of health authorities to Parliament was correct. As a response to that criticism the review process represents a significant step forward in improving both the accountability and the quality of the plans themselves. In addition, the review forum provides Ministers and RHAs with an opportunity to exchange views on the problems, difficulties and priorities facing the NHS. How the process will be used will obviously depend to a large extent on the managerial style of Ministers. An autocratic approach will probably result in a monologue from Ministers and prevent a constructive exchange. If this occurs, the review process could become limited in its value.

4.5   The NHS Planning System

The starting point is the strategic plans which have to be prepared by DHAs after referring to the RHAs strategic planning guidelines. Where a ten-year strategy has already been prepared this will provide the base for the RHAs' strategic planning guidelines. These will be derived from a review of the previous regional strategy, taking account of subsequent achievements and events. This exercise will culminate in the issue of specific RHA strategic planning guidelines for each DHA which should reflect national priorities as they relate to the region. Where existing strategies do not exist, the RHA is expected to formulate strategic planning guidelines in collaboration with DHAs.

The next step is for each DHA to prepare its strategic plan within the RHAs' guidelines. One significant aspect of these strategic planning guidelines, for District Treasurers, is the information relating to the resource assumptions; revenue, capital and manpower. Forecasts of revenue and capital usually include the estimated effects of future inflation and it is not easy to readily identify any projected growth or contraction of finance. However the real changes in revenue and capital must be estimated in order to prepare strategic plans. The resource base of each DHA strategic plan has important consequences for the pace of its implementation and a careful assessment of the degree of optimism or pessimism reflected in the forecasts is essential. Regional Treasurers may have undertaken a similar assessment of the assumptions provided by the DHSS, and adjusted these to reflect their view of the financial, economic and political future. District Treasurers will need to consider the likely resource base of the DHA so that they can advise their fellow chief officers, and eventually the DHA, of the scope for development or the need for retrenchment. The assessment of future resources is a complex task influenced by many factors such as the Government's policy, but is clearly one of crucial importance if planning is to be effective. Consequently, in Chapter 7 we have discussed how such resource forecasts for revenue and capital may be prepared.

Having examined and accepted or modified the resource assumptions for revenue and capital, the District Treasurer can turn his attention to the manpower assumptions included in the RHA's strategic guidelines. In order to assess their realism, these assumptions, have to be scrutinised carefully. This is especially important because, in general, manpower forecasts in the NHS are not soundly based, due to the extreme difficulty of obtaining a national or regional picture from reliable local data. For example, recruitment prospects of medical staff vary greatly between parts of the country according to the desirability of residing in a particular area. Consequently, care must be taken when applying national or regional manpower assumptions in the local context and DHAs must exercise their discretion. However, one aspect remains dominant, the projected size of the DHAs potential labour force should be related to revenue assumptions and manpower targets. This should include an assessment of the extent to which the required supply of the additional appropriate manpower can be

financed from future development additions. If the additional manpower
requirements can not be financed, or exceed manpower targets then a more
difficult task must be undertaken. The DHA must decide if the resources
can be released from other sources, such as existing levels of service and
failing this, it will have to reconsider its manpower policy.

Manpower represents the largest element of real resources of the NHS,
and is therefore at least as important an element of a strategic plan as the
capital and revenue elements. If a DHA or RHA strategic plan is to have any
real value, it must be described, defined and stated in manpower terms. The
advantages of this approach are that the financial implications can be
readily assessed from the manpower information and more importantly
can be easily controlled. If the resource assumptions turn out to be inaccurate, which, because of their nature, is more than likely, then the adjustments
to the strategy can be effected in terms of manpower resources.

A further aspect of the DHAs strategic plan is the commentary on major
service deficiencies or imbalances, and, most significantly, the areas in
which the national or regional policies do not seem to be appropriate or are
being ignored. Each DHA is given the opportunity to explain and justify
any stance which ignores DHSS priorities. While this seems to recognise
apparent weaknesses in the planning system, it also has the advantage of
directing the RHAs attention to the main matters of the strategy.

Eventually, the strategic plans will be agreed, at least in most cases. They
can then form the basis of each DHAs annual programme which sets out
the DHAs proposals for the next two years. The general principle is that
these plans should be consistent with the corresponding years of the agreed
strategy after taking account of the revised resource assumptions provided
by the DHSS or the RHA, as appropriate. They should include an action
plan for the next financial year and a programme for the second year.

These proposals should incorporate two important features. One is a
capital programme for the coming year which shows the minor items of
capital expenditure coming under the control of the DHA. The other is a
revenue budget for the next financial year. The main implication for the
District Treasurer is that these two elements of the plan are to be based on
the revised resource assumptions and presented to the DHA. The job will be
made easier if the strategic plan is supported by a ten-year capital and
revenue programme. The appropriate year of this programme can then be
quickly modified as necessary and incorporated into the operational plan.

As this ten-year programme is itself a product of speculation on future
resources, contingency programmes based on alternative resource
assumptions would help the transposition of the programme into the shorter
two year timescale.

4.6 The NHS Planning System in Action

In an organisational setting, the ideas of planning and control are often seen as part of a continuous cycle. It is sometimes theoretically described as a series of events in which the planning system begins with setting priorities, and results in feedback which can modify the original priorities. The merit of such an approach has been recorded as being rational and results in a well structured approach to the management task of choosing between priorities. It also recognises that planning is a series of discrete but related events and that appropriate techniques and expertise can be enlisted at various stages.

Finding such a process actually in operation may be an impossible quest. In practice, the distinction between the events may become blurred. For example, setting priorities can be divorced from the planning system. In addition, selected priorities may often be reactionary expedients and more radical and perhaps appropriate options may never be devised. While theorists may be critical of the more limited approach of practitioners, it can be legitimately argued that the practitioner's style is both pragmatic and well suited to their particular needs and environment.

So it is in the NHS. The theoretical cycle does not exist unmodified. In practice, the NHS Planning System tends to be an instrument of control in that it is used to ensure that RHAs and DHAs conform to DHSS priorities in broad terms. This modified NHS management cycle has two separate parts. First, fixing priorities, which is the role of the DHSS, is a 'top down' approach isolated from the NHS Planning System. The DHSS develops its preferred priorities for the NHS from both its own assessment of needs and the value-judgements of the Secretary of State. The aggregated priorities of the RHAs and DHAs do not feature directly in this process. Instead, these are reflected in the other part of the cycle, the NHS Planning System. This attempts to establish and demonstrate that the RHAs' interpretation of DHSS priorities is reflected in DHAs' strategic plans and annual programme and that DHAs will implement national priorities within their financial allocations.

Turning priorities into action can be dependent on many variables. The two most significant are likely to be linked; the first is the commitment to the priorities and the second is related to the resources available at the time of implementation. Commitment to priorities may be related to the degree of participation in their formulation. As already mentioned, RHAs and DHAs tend not to participate effectively in the formation of NHS priorities in a way that allows them to put forward a view of their specific, directly assessed requirements. If local priorities have eventually to be subordinated to national priorities over the long term, the local priorities are likely to assume a much greater significance to RHAs and DHAs in the short term. When demands on limited current resources are being considered by RHAs and DHAs, they may tend to favour their own local priorities where these differ from those of the DHSS. Temptation with opportunity is unlikely to be resisted and the financial aspects of the NHS Planning System can provide the opportunity as we now explain.

Assumptions about future years capital and revenue allocations form the major part of the resource base for the NHS Planning System. Because of their nature, they are not usually highly accurate. Small, but marginally significant, variations occur each year which are not forecast precisely and in fact are difficult to predict. For example, July of 1983/84 saw an arbitary real cut of 1% in the national revenue allocation. Such unpredictable changes in the resource base, which are a result of the Government's fiscal, monetary and economic policy, create a degree of uncertainty for DHAs, which give them the opportunity to justify deferring national priorities.

The precise effect cannot be measured by the performance review such as those of the DHSS or RHA. Scope exists for DHAs to slip in local priorities and still be able to demonstrate that the actual effect of deferring national priorities is due entirely to imposed resource constraints. This can be shown by linking the ostensible commitment to priorities with financial limitations. In this way, local opportunities for service developments, which may arise without warning, can be grasped by a DHA.

The scope for such divergence can be gauged from the history of the allocation for interim secure units. Since the mid-seventies, the DHSS has allocated monies to the RHAs in order to stimulate the programme for the provision of secure units for mentally-ill offenders. One was to be provided in each of the 14 regions in England. The allocations were made in advance of the necessary spending to act as a catalyst, and were made available without adequate control over the provision of the facilities. Constitution-ally, if health authorities were unable to spend the money, they were to hold the money in reserve pending the appointed day. A more accurate view of what has happened is that the money has been diverted to finance other locally assessed priorities, often not even associated with mentally-ill offenders. The Comptroller and Auditor General are now beginning to question how the money has been used, but long after the health authorities have diverted the resources.

It is to overcome such loose ends of the planning system that the Reviews were introduced, as we mentioned in section 4.4. The question to be asked is: *Does the review process actually achieve its goal?* The answer is not clear yet. One difficulty in gauging its success is the limited experience of only one annual round of reviews. These suffered severely from limited information on important matters such as performance indicators and therefore any fair assessment must recognise these initial limitations.

What can be said is that most, if not all, health authorities took the first round extremely seriously. This in itself can be seen as a recognition both of the importance of the approach and the relevance of the issues and topics explored. Several pertinent questions were raised on issues such as under-utilised resources, unsolved problems and unimplemented priorities and in this respect the reviews were used to identify matters of significance and can be considered as successful.

One major weakness of the reviews is the lack of sound information on performance and in particular costs. The cost information that is readily available is that published in the annual cost booklets. These are not current unit costs in the commercial dynamic sense but the total annual expenditure of each service divided by the various units of service such as in-patient days. Such a crude unit of expenditure is not adequate for precise and detailed performance reviews and new and improved systems are required before the reviews can be judged as successful in this respect. Work is already in hand to attempt to improve measures of throughput and it is now up to Treasurers to respond constructively and extend these into reliable unit costs as used by many other businesses including the private health sector. We have discussed costing in greater detail in Chapter 8.

Again in the context of measuring the success of the reviews, identifying such weaknesses in the information available to management is of value in itself. How the NHS responds is another matter. One important feature of these problems is that they related mainly to the question of efficient use of resources. Where the review process was successful was that health authorities had to explain and justify any lack of progress in implementing agreed priorities. Such a dialogue did in fact provide the previously missing feedback of the NHS Planning System. The signs for future reviews are even more encouraging in that health authorities are likely to be put under increasing pressure to make progress towards national priorities. Given that the Secretary of State is constitutionally responsible for the NHS this aspect of the review process is clearly successful and valid.

One major implication for planning in the NHS is not often acknowledged. While the role and responsibilities of DHAs are set out the question arises as to the appropriateness of the size of many DHAs to carry out the task effectively. If they are too small to be an effective planning unit then the RHA will be the natural agent to assume the role. In this respect RHAs could become the effective planning unit for the NHS and such an outcome seems more likely with the additional influence given to RHAs by the review process.

'Care in Action' sets out the Government's guidance for DHAs on national priorities for the health and personal social services. The Government's declared role is seen as being to promulgate and monitor national priorities, modifying them as necessary in the light of authorities' experience. However, as already mentioned, little account tends to be taken of DHA's experience in modifying national priorities.

'Care in Action' included an open letter from the Secretary of State, to the chairmen and members of DHAs. This acknowledged that the handbook merely set out the main priorities which DHAs should follow in running their services, while simultaneously recognising the scope for DHAs to pursue their own priorities, by giving them as much freedom as possible to decide how to pursue the Government's priorities.

The extent of this apparent contradiction between central promulgation of priorities and local freedom can be established by further advice, again provided by the Secretary of State. He indicated that DHAs have a wider opportunity than their predecessors to plan and develop services in the light of local needs and circumstances while having regard to national priorities.

The former health authorities were asked to take account of such national priorities and shift resources from the more glamorous work of the NHS, such as surgery and medicine, to the 'cinderella services', like those for the elderly and mentally handicapped. However, presumably after assessing their local needs, they did not seem to comply. It has been shown, that the priorities laid down by the Government in March 1976 in the consultative document 'Priorities for the Health and Personal Social Services in England' required a shift in resources between the services for the various patient groups. The shift was not implemented and the lack of co-operation was attributed to the power of the medical staff in the NHS to determine the distribution of resources between patient groups. In particular it was concluded that senior hospital doctors, who provide acute services, have more influence in the distribution of resources than those doctors who provide caring services for long-stay patients. This outcome arose even when priorities were fairly precisely defined in a document which specified the desired distribution of resources between the patient groups. The current broader priorities will elicit even less conviction if DHAs so choose to interpret the required redistribution of resources to its favour.

Not all of 'Care in Action' is of such limited value. Where it does improve on the previous documents is its resource base. National priorities are set firmly in the context of a realistic view of future resources of finance and manpower. Realistic at this time means limited growth, as included in the PESC review and consequently, 'Care in Action' recognises and accepts that the redistribution of resources will be a slow process over a long period. This view of the future is the justification for not setting targets for the resources to be allocated to each patient group.

Having no pre-set measurable target makes effective monitoring extremely difficult. The Government seems to have fixed its role in NHS planning as that of a prompter in the wings and as a result has no authority to prevent DHAs from slipping in their own ad libs. While this has been the case for many years, and attempts since 1974 have not changed the position, the Government is clearly putting its faith in the review process.

4.7   The Role of the RHAs in the NHS Planning System

The RHAs are the agents of the DHSS in controlling priorities. They are interposed between the DHSS and the DHAs in the NHS Planning System and their role could be crucial to the effectiveness and success of the implementation of national priorities. Their first task is to encourage DHAs to effect the changes in services required to achieve the national priorities. At first glance, there does not seem to be much hope for success, in this respect, by merely adding another exhorting voice to the utterings of the DHSS. However, RHAs have a powerful weapon in their persuasive armoury which can support their aims, namely their role in allocating resources, particularly revenue. While this function is already an accepted role of RHAs, it assumes greater significance when it is seen as influencing priorities. In Chapter 6 we have outlined an approach to resource allocation which can be used to persuade DHAs to conform to national aims. However, such an approach conflicts with the main and officially designated role of resource allocation in the NHS, which is to achieve geographic equality in the availability of comparable services. When the alternatives of geographic equality and a preferred distribution of resources between patient groups are considered, the DHSS practice has consistently been to give greater emphasis to geographic equality. Capital and revenue monies are distributed to RHAs on this basis through the RAWP mechanism and modified, but related, approaches are used by most RHAs to allocate revenue to DHAs.

The power of the revenue allocation is already well known. It has been tried and tested in many parts of the public sector, and can be even more influential in the NHS where DHAs rely almost entirely on Government finance. As we said previously, before the RAWP methodology was used, additional revenue was earmarked to specific developments, such as new hospitals. Such a link can still be maintained so that general financial growth can be used to direct DHAs towards the priorities promulgated by the DHSS. If additional revenue is dependent on particular proposals, then the RHA has a much easier task to monitor policy. For example, it is much easier to see if a service to geriatrics is expanded by an agreed number of nurses and beds than to monitor a shift in resources in financial terms, which is probably based on very broad potentially unreliable estimates.

As we describe later, the analysis of spending by client groups is not a carefully structured accounting matter, but a broad apportionment of spending to groups. This includes many assumptions. For example, dividing the cost of a DGH between the types of patients is not a direct result of patient costing systems, but an assumption of the type that say 50% of the patients would absorb 50% of the cost. This is clearly too broad compared to the physical analysis of beds and manpower. The non financial data may be more helpful and appropriate when RHAs are monitoring the use of additional resources.

Managing the region's capital programme is the other significant role of RHAs in the Planning System. In this, RHAs again have the opportunity to direct capital towards their preferred priorities. While capital monies are committed for some years ahead, it is relatively easy to change direction on the priorities to be pursued by capital allocations over the longer time scale envisaged with the NHS Planning System. However, effective capital deployment depends, to a large degree, on the availability of revenue monies to finance the additional running costs, and this balance requires careful attention. If RHAs encourage a particular deployment of capital, the DHAs may not be able to support the consequential deployment of revenue, and it is in this respect that the RHA has another major role.

Before agreeing to a regional strategy, the RHA must be satisfied that it is financially feasible. Resource projections, both for the region as a whole and each DHA must be completed carefully, while DHA strategies based on those forecasts must be considered with care, to ensure that the capital and revenue requirements are attainable. It is of limited value to proceed with a multi-million pound hospital development to realise later that the DHA will have insufficient revenue, or that the revenue required will be so great as to preclude priorities of other DHAs. This task requires a change of emphasis in RHAs, which in many regions has already begun.

The former RCCS revenue allocations were capital led. The allocation of revenue was therefore dependent on the allocation of capital. This approach needs to be adjusted to reflect the view that both capital and revenue resources should be given similar weight in planning health services. The RHA is charged with the role of achieving such a balance.

Opportunities for RHAs to influence DHAs plans are provided at frequent intervals in the NHS Planning System. As mentioned previously, they start the ball rolling by issuing planning guidelines to DHAs, after consultation with them. Subsequently the RHA has to be available to discuss any difficulties that DHAs encounter while preparing their plans, and more specifically, have to meet DHAs regularly to review and discuss both strategic plans and annual programmes. These are probably the most significant events for RHAs. They can discuss, negotiate, plead, exhort, threaten or act in any appropriate way to persuade DHAs to conform to national/regional priorities.

Alternatively, DHAs have the opportunity to explain why they should not. It is in this forum that the RHAs are faced with a choice. After considering the DHAs view of local needs and aggregating these into a regional view, the RHA may decide that the local priorities may be more urgent than those of the DHSS. Such a position for RHAs may arise because of the greater freedom now allowed to DHAs to plan and develop their services. While RHAs may often find themselves continuing to support the DHSS advice, any support for a contrary regional view arising from the aggregation of the DHAs priorities could result in the RHA having to disagree with DHSS guidance. The RHA would then find itself in a position with the DHSS which resembles that between the DHA and the RHA. So it can be seen that the RHA can either act as the expression of the DHAs views on priorities and attempt to restructure national priorities, or it can adopt national priorities and attempt to restructure DHAs priorities. Its role is one of influence based on the interface of national and local priorities.

The NHS Planning System provides for regular meetings between the DHAs, the RHAs and the DHSS. On these occasions strategic plans and annual programmes can be reviewed and any divergence between the parties can obviously be considered. While the DHSS may have greater authority, and give RHAs the opportunity to plead special cases, the RHAs influence as 'pig in the middle' is potentially extensive. It could also suffer from ambivalence. *Will it act as DHSS agent or DHA spokesman? Perhaps both at different times?* It is possible that because of a lack of consistency in a RHAs role, its interposition between the DHSS and DHAs may weaken the RHAs influence to such an extent, that again DHAs may have the opportunity to pursue their own priorities.

5

Financial Control and Accountability of the National Health Service

5.1 The Approach

In Chapter 3 we discussed how monies are allocated by Government to individual RHAs, which in turn allocate resources to the DHAs. Since the Government finances the NHS it is clear that it is not going to allow health authorities a completely free hand in how they conduct their affairs. The Government's interest is likely to have two aspects. First there is control, whereby Government uses certain powers to control particular activities of health authorities and in this chapter we shall examine what form of financial control is imposed by Government. In reality the financial control exercised is very powerful, but also rather crude, namely the power to decide the amount of money that can be spent by each RHA. In a similar manner the RHA can exert control over the DHA, as it controls a DHA's level of funds. Control over the spending of health authorities is exercised by means of the cash limit system, which will be discussed in the first part of this chapter.

Secondly, health authorities are accountable to the Secretary of State for their actions and consequently are required to report to him at the end of each financial year. One way in which this accountability is discharged is by the production of annual financial accounts and statements. We shall describe the nature of these accounts and statements and then offer an explanation of why they fail to discharge, satisfactorily, the duty of accountability.

Linked to the production of annual accounts and statements are the activities of the external auditor. In most organisations, once accounts have been prepared, it is usual for them to be examined by an independent auditor, who will attest to their accuracy and reliability. This is the job of the external auditor and the NHS is something of an exception to the rule in that it has not one but two forms of external audit. One is the audit undertaken by an auditor working for the DHSS, the other is the audit duty carried out by the staff of the National Audit Office directed by the Comptroller and Auditor General.

5.2   The Cash Limit System

In Chapter 3 we noted that the allocation of funds to the NHS, in total, and to individual health authorities, is cash limited. Since 1976 the cash limit has become of great importance to Governments in their attempts to control the level of public expenditure and, while the cash limit approach can be said to be 'politically' successful, there are drawbacks in its operation. Although, in practice, the cash limit system is very complex, it is fundamentally a very simple concept and we shall attempt here to describe the logic and method of its approach.

As we have already seen, the legal authorisation to incur public expenditure is given by Parliament, via the Estimates Procedure. Prior to 1976/77, in voting funds to a particular programme, such as health or defence, the assumption was that Parliament was authorising an amount of public expenditure that was to be constant in real terms. By 'constant in real terms' we mean that the approved expenditure each year would pay for the same amount of goods and services, such as materials or manpower, whatever the ruling level of pay and prices. If there was any inflation in the economy, then clearly the only way in which public expenditure could be maintained in real or volume terms was by the voting of additional funds to cover that increased cost due to inflation. This was, in fact, what happened. Periodically, the Treasury would request Parliament to vote additional sums, by means of a Supplementary Estimate, to cover the effects of inflation. This procedure was virtually open-ended and whatever the inflationary increases in pay and prices, additional funds would be voted to cover the effects. A simplified illustration of this procedure is shown in Table 6 overleaf.

For many years these procedures were regarded as being quite satisfactory. While rates of inflation were very low, at levels such as 2-3% per annum, the sums voted in Supplementary Estimates were small, relative to total public expenditure. However, in 1974/75 the British economy began to suffer extremely high rates of inflation and consequently, because of its open-ended nature, the large sums voted in Supplementary Estimates assumed a new significance. The allegation was often made that public expenditure was out of control and something should be done. Something was in fact done; cash limits were introduced.

Basically, what the cash limit does is to restrain the amount of cash spent on Government programmes. Instead of the open-ended funding of inflation by means of Supplementary Estimates, the Treasury now places a limit

Table 6 — Illustration of Supplementary Estimates

	£000
1,000 employees at a salary of £6,000 p.s.	6,000
15,000 tons of materials at £1,000 per ton	15,000
Initial Vote	21,000

After six months of the year suppose the following pay and price increases have occurred:-

a) Wage rates by 5%
b) Material costs by 5%

To maintain public expenditure in volume terms, namely 1,000 employees and 15,000 tons, additional finance must be made available by means of a Supplementary Estimate:-

	£000
Wages = £6 million x 5% p.a. x 6 months	150
Materials = £15 million x 5% p.a. x 6 months	375
Supplementary Estimate	525

on the amount of additional finance it will request from Parliament. Under this cash limit approach, Parliament will vote a Supplementary Estimate based on the Treasury's forecast of inflation in the coming year. The Main Estimate, combined with the Supplementary Estimate, is termed the cash limit and this is the limit on spending irrespective of what the actual rates of inflation turn out to be. So, if the Treasury's estimate of inflation was 5%, this was incorporated in the cash limit and if actual inflation turned out to be 10%, Government departments and the NHS would still have to live within their cash limits. In most cases this would mean reducing the level of expenditure in volume terms. Cash limits apply to some 60% of public spending, and while our description is necessarily simple, it provides the essence of the cash limits approach. Before discussing the effects of cash limits on health authorities we first wish to make a few points about cash limits in general.

a. Volume versus Cash

The defect in the control of public expenditure prior to cash limits was that while Parliament, via the Treasury, was able to control the volume of public expenditure, the amount of cash disbursements was open-ended and hence not controlled. With the cash limit approach the whole method has been turned around. Although the amount of cash is now being controlled, the volume of public expenditure is not. Parliament initially votes a certain volume of public expenditure, but the actual volume of expenditure depends on how close the actual rate of inflation is to the forecast. If actual inflation is greater than forecast, then the volume of public expenditure will be less than that originally authorised by Parliament, and vice-versa.

b. Hidden Cuts in Services

Cash limits have been used by governments to produce hidden cuts in resources, in a clandestine manner. Consider the NHS as an example. In 1982/83 the Secretary of State was not able to increase the cash limits to finance all of the cost of pay awards and announced that part of the development addition would be used for that purpose. In such circumstances one can only assume that this deliberate underfunding of inflation was designed to engineer a cutback in services since the planned growth in resources was reduced by the underfunding of inflation.

To be fair, it should be mentioned that shortfalls in the funding of inflation may subsequently be made up, partially or fully, in the cash limit of the following year, but this does not alter the fact that the effect of underfunding during the current year is a cut in services.

c. Surrogate Incomes Policy

Although Governments of all political complexions declare their opposition to incomes policy, at least for a time, they often tend to introduce it in some form or another. The cash limit for NHS staff costs was set at 3% for 1984/85 and clearly this was intended to signal to those involved in wage bargaining that the Government wished to see pay settlements of around 3% for that year. Thus the cash limit approach can be regarded as a surrogate for an incomes policy, at least for the public sector.

5.3   Cash Limits and the NHS

As the NHS comprises a large part of the public sector, cash limits obviously have a major impact on health authorities. Initially, the DHSS is required to contain total NHS spending but excluding FPCs, within two cash limits: one for capital and one for revenue. These are approved by Parliament and translated by the DHSS into cash limits for each RHA. The DHSS then requires the RHAs to contain their spending within the cash limits provided. The RHA will then set cash limits for each of its DHAs, and DHAs in turn are required to contain their spending within their own cash limits. FPC expenditure is a demand-based service, and as such is not subject to the constraints of cash limits.

The first point of confusion concerns what exactly a health authority's cash limit really means. It will be recalled that cash limits refer to the level of disbursements from the National Exchequer. Individual health authorities obtain funds from the DHSS for transfer into their own bank accounts. In very broad terms, a health authority's revenue cash limit is a limit on the amount of money that can be requisitioned from the DHSS in any one year. It is not a limit on the actual expenditure of the authority. The difference between the health authority's expenditure and the level of funds requisitioned consists of the changes in the balances of current assets and liabilities. These include the balances of cash in the health authority's bank account and the levels of stocks, debtors and creditors. Changes in these balances can distort the health authority's cash limit in a single year. The effect can be quite pronounced. It is worth describing here, in order to demonstrate the restricted approach to financial control offered by cash limits.

Let us consider a fictitious DHA. At the beginning of the financial year it has a bank balance of £100,000. It is then given a cash limit of £40 million. If the DHA can reduce its bank balance to nil by the end of the financial year, it will have available to spend its cash limit of £40 million plus its bank balance of £100,000: a total of £40.1 million.

Similarly, changes in the other balances can be managed to generate cash. For example, an increase in the DHA's creditors between the beginning and end of the financial year will mean that bills will be paid in the following financial year, thus reducing the demands on the current year's cash limits. So it is with a decrease in the DHA's debtors; more cash will have been collected. In addition, stocks can be run down, so reducing the goods to be paid for in a financial year.

The arrangements for capital cash limits are slightly different in that they are concerned more with the actual payments made during the financial year. Furthermore, the scope for adjusting capital cash limits by changes in balances tends to be more limited than for the revenue cash limit.

What happens if a health authority, for some reason or another, cannot meet its cash limit? In the case of a health authority which exceeds its revenue cash limit, the usual penalty is that the overspending will be deducted from its allocation for the following financial year. In this situation the authority will probably need to take action to ensure that it does not exceed its cash limit in the following year as well. It is illegal for health authorities to over-spend, and while it may be tolerated by the DHSS for one year, persistent overspending may result in legal action.

If an authority underspends its revenue cash limit then not all of the underspent funds are lost to it. The DHSS permits RHAs to carry forward up to 1% of its revenue cash limit into the following year. Similarly under-spending on capital can be carried forward. However, these carry forward provisions have frequently been criticised by District Treasurers as being inadequate, but in the present financial climate it seems unlikely that a more generous carry forward will be permitted. It should also be noted that health authorities have limited powers to transfer sums between their revenue and capital cash limits. RHAs have the power to transfer up to 1% of revenue funds to capital and up to 10% of capital funds to revenue. Furthermore, it should be mentioned that the RHA may authorise greater carry-forwards and transfers to individual DHAs, providing that the over-all regional constraints on the RHA's cash limits for capital and revenue are not exceeded without the Secretary of State's approval.

What then are the results of applying this system of cash limits to health authority finances? The first point we would make is that, contrary to what is frequently stated, the various aspects of the cash limit do enable the health authority Treasurer to have some financial flexibility. Within the limits laid down the following factors can be controlled:

(a) transfer between revenue and capital
(b) utilisation of the carry-forward provisions to adjust the effective cash limit for the year
(c) adjusting balances to influence the actual level of cash available in the current year while remaining within the cash limit.

These three factors combined give the Treasurer scope to influence the actual level of spending in the financial year.

Secondly, cash limits can result in an inefficient use of resources. Most health service staff are familiar with year-end spending sprees, when a potential underspending has been identified and consequently, these funds suddenly become freely available for single items of equipment, maintenance work and the like. This phenomenon has been referred to as the 'Treasurer's January sales'. While not much real waste is likely to occur, it is frequently the case that those responsible for specific services will purchase equipment that is not their first choice, but is all they can buy and pay for in the time available. We accept that this is not really a consequence of the cash limit itself but of the limited carry forward of funds permitted and perhaps poor budgeting. Indeed the evidence available appears to indicate that this year-end spending spree is now less prominent than it used to be as a result of the introduction of limited carry forward facilities. Furthermore, many Treasurers are aware that given good financial management, year-end spending sprees can be avoided even with the present limited carry forward.

Thirdly, the cash limits system represents a constraint on the financial resources of each health authority. While the cash limits can be adjusted to a degree, after any adjustment has been effected, they are still a constraint on the amount of cash available. In this respect they are not a constructive method of financial control. They make no attempt to influence the way in which cash is spent, what it is spent on, or how effectively it is used. Cash limits are mainly concerned with the amount of cash drawn from the National Exchequer. In order to exert control on this level of spending, the DHSS monitors the NHS cash position both regularly and frequently. The mechanism is part of the DHSS financial information system (FIS). We have outlined this in the following section.

5.4   Financial Information System (FIS)

FIS is mainly a reporting system which requires every health athority to submit regular financial returns to the DHSS. Some returns, for example those relating to pay awards and the volume of health authority spending, are submitted annually. Others are submitted much more frequently, and most of these relate to the cash limit system. It is to these that we turn in this section.

The FIS returns form part of the DHSS financial control over the NHS. Each has a different purpose and we have briefly described their role in the control process.

The main functions of these FIS returns are to enable the DHSS to monitor the progress of a DHA in managing its cash limits. One FIS return declares the DHA's cash limits after adjusting for over- and under-spending brought forward and any transfers between capital and revenue. Subsequent FIS returns show the cash requisitioned to date plus a forecast for the remainder of the year for each cash limit. Other FIS returns deal with the level of health authority's bank balances and provide information about FPCs.

Health authority cash requisitions are submitted to the DHSS weekly and specify the cash advances required for each day in the week ahead plus an estimate of the total of the three subsequent weeks. The cash so advanced does not meet all the expenses of the health authority, as some payments, such as the employer's national insurance contributions are made centrally by the DHSS. This return provides the DHSS with limited information about each DHA's cash requirements rather than the cash limit position in total. A slightly different emphasis is given to this return compared to the other FIS returns. From December to March of each year, DHAs also have to submit this return to the RHA. If the DHSS gauge that a particular cash advance will seriously exceed the region's overall cash limit, then the RHA will be advised so that necessary action can be taken. It is at this stage that the monitoring process can turn into control. The RHAs have the opportunity to influence events rather than observe them. However, in reality, the RHAs seldom, if ever, exert such control, as the consequences tend to be far-reaching. Imagine the situation where an offending DHA has by February already spent its cash limit. If the RHA steps in and prevents an overspending by refusing to advance any more cash, the DHA would be unable to pay its wages or creditors. The RHA would effectively be bankrupting the DHA. The less traumatic alternative is to advance the cash and penalise the DHA by deducting the overspending from future cash limits. So the exertion of financial control is retrospective.

This rather complex financial reporting mechanism has been included in our chapter on financial control because it is seen by the DHSS as contributing to the financial control of the NHS. As we have described, the information collected is used primarily to record what has occurred or is expected to occur. We consider this to be closer to monitoring rather than control, as the latter implies that corrective action will arise where the information does not accord with expectations.

5.5   Statutory Annual Accounts and Statements

Nearly all types of organisation in both the private and public sector are required by law to produce some sort of financial accounts and statements at the end of each financial year. For example, limited companies are required to produce final accounts according to the requirements of the Companies Act while local authorities prepare accounts according to a format prescribed by the Secretary of State for the Environment. The rationale for producing these financial accounts and statements is that they should provide sufficient information to enable interested persons to understand and make decisions about the organisation. It is usually difficult to decide what kind of information is most relevant to these persons but as far as the public sector is concerned, we suggest that one major information need involves accountability. Each year health authorities use public monies to run their services and must be held accountable for the use of these monies. One way of achieving such accountability is by the production of annual financial accounts and statements showing how funds have been utilised. The conventional way of producing such financial statements is as follows:

(a) income and expenditure account
(b) balance sheet.

The income and expenditure account summarises the financial trans-actions of the organisation during the past year. It adopts the accruals concept which dictates that the expenditure included reflects the cost of goods and services consumed during the year, rather than the amount paid for. Similarly the income shown is that actually earned rather than cash received during the year. Income earned but not received is classified as debtors. In the NHS, income and expenditure accounts are prepared on this accounting convention, but with one major difference: health authorities do not include an annual charge for dep-reciation of assets. This would reflect the wear and tear of items, such as equipment and buildings, which could be reasonably charged in a par-ticular financial year. This omission of depreciation is because health authorities do not account for capital assets according to usual accounting conventions, as we explain later.

The balance sheet in most organisations shows the financial position as at the end of the year in terms of assets and liabilities. The assets may consist of current assets such as cash, stock and debtors, and capital assets such as land, buildings and equipment. On the liability side will be shown current liabilities, such as creditors, and also items such as loans out-standing and the owner's share in the business. The capital assets are usually shown at a written-down cost, as a result of a depreciation charge being made each year to reflect the wear and tear of these assets. An appreciation in assets such as land and buildings may be included.

Health authority balance sheets, however, do not conform to conven-tional accounting practice in that they only show current assets and current liabilities such as its bank balance, creditor and debtor balances and stocks. Capital assets and liabilities are not shown in health authorities' balance sheets as the NHS is not required to record the value of its capital assets such as buildings and land. A health authority balance sheet thus shows limited information.

One major problem of the annual accounts and statements of the NHS as a whole is their accounting consistency. The annual accounts for the NHS are compiled by aggregating the annual accounts of all DHAs and RHAs, together with those for centrally provided services. However, there is a considerable variation in accounting practice between health authorities. For example, one health authority may price its stores issues by using an average price of all like items in stock, while another may use the price assuming that the first item brought into stores is the first item issued. Such a difference in accounting practice will mean that an item included in one DHA's accounts will be priced at a different amount compared to that in another DHA's accounts. The implication of different accounting practices being applied in the NHS is that the aggregated NHS accounts become less valuable and appropriate for the purpose of accountability. Improvements in accounting practice and standards are currently being considered in the NHS.

The precise format of the annual accounts and statements of health authorities is fixed by the DHSS and can in fact vary slightly between years. Broadly speaking three kinds of analysis are prepared:-

a.   Functional Accounts

This shows the expenditure of the health authority classified according to broad function. Examples are hospital services and community services. Both capital and revenue expenditure are analysed in this way.

b.   Subjective Accounts

This classifies health authority expenditure according to its nature. Examples include medical salaries, nursing salaries, drugs, dressings and provisions. The main subjective analysis is in relation to revenue expenditure, and more limited analysis is included for capital expenditure.

c.   Annual Statements

These include a statement of the cash drawn from the DHSS, both capital and revenue, together with a reconciliation with the net expenditure. Other miscellaneous items are dealt with in these statements, such as the losses and compensation payments approved by the health authority during the year.

5.6   Costing Returns

In addition to the annual accounts and statements health authorities also provide additional costing information. For each of their hospitals, they are asked to produce a variety of information such as cost per in-patient day and cost per out-patient day. In addition, costing information is produced for community service and support services such as catering. These costs returns can be used in a number of ways, but their main value is for comparative purposes, whereby one DHA can compare its hospital costs with other DHAs. There are, however, several drawbacks to the use of such returns. For one thing, there is a considerable element of inconsist-

ency as regards the accounting principles used in their preparation and so
DHAs may prepare them in different ways. This would clearly reduce the
value of any comparative exercise between DHAs. Also a considerable
time elapses between the end of a financial year and the publication of the
cost returns, especially the DHSS/Regional summaries and consequently
the information is rather obsolete when it is published. More is said about
this in Chapter 8.

5.7   Accountability

Several points need to be made about the purpose and utility of these
statutory returns. At the end of the financial year, health authorities
commit a considerable amount of staff time in preparing these accounts
and statements and therefore it is desirable that they are of some use.
Although we know of no definitive evidence as to what groups of people
would make use of health authority accounts, it is interesting to speculate
that the following either do or might make use of such accounts:

(a) health authority members
(b) health authority employees
(c) trade unions
(d) local authorities
(e) community health councils
(f) the DHSS
(g) Public Accounts Committee.

Accounting theory dictates that the main criterion for producing information in public accounts is its usefulness to users in making decisions and
this criterion applies as much to a health authority as to any other
organisation. If the present accounts and statements do not meet the needs
of users then logically they should be discarded and replaced with something else. It could be argued, however, that since the detailed format of the
accounts is laid down by the major user group, namely the DHSS, then the
correct type of accounting information is already being produced.

Presumably the main reason for producing health authority accounts is
that, after consolidation for the NHS as a whole, they provide the main
vehicle for accountability to Parliament. We suggest however, that there
are some defects in the type of accounting information shown in health
authority statutory accounts. These can be summarised as follows:

a Planning Versus Reporting

As has been seen earlier, planning in the NHS is performed on the basis of client groups whereby decisions are made about the allocation of resources between the different segments of the population. These are referred to as client groups. It will be noted that the financial accounts make no reference to client groups. No attempt is made to show how resources have actually been committed between client groups and this appears to us to be a major weakness. It seems illogical for health authorities to prepare plans on the basis of client groups and then to report progress in terms of spending on a completely different basis. This is exemplified below in Figure 5.

Figure 5 - Illustration of Planning and Financial Reporting

PLANNING – on the basis of client group	FINANCIAL REPORTING – on the basis of subjective/objective analysis	
	Subjective	Objective
Geriatric	Medical Costs	Hospitals
Mentally Ill	Nursing Costs	Community
Mentally Handicapped	Drugs	Administration
etc.	Provisions, etc.	

b Effectiveness and Efficiency

Health authority accounts give no indication of how effectively and efficiently resources have been used. They merely show how much has been spent and the items of expenditure. While it is easy to be critical of this lack of information, it is considerably more difficult, if not impossible, to devise such measures for the purposes of accountability. This is mainly due to the problems of measuring the output of health services.

5.8 Voluntary Reporting

Although health authorities are obliged by statute to produce that accounting information required by Parliament, there is nothing to prevent them providing additional information where they feel this would be useful. Such voluntary reports would be primarily aimed at locally based user groups and would have the advantage that the information shown would be:

(a) More relevant to local user groups
(b) In a more readable and comprehensible format

A recent publication by the Chartered Institute of Public Finance and Accountancy (CIPFA) has discussed such voluntary reporting by health authorities and has made suggestions about the sort of information that might be included. Some examples are:

(a) Spending by client group
(b) Spending comparisons between years
(c) Reconciliation between accounts and cash limits
(d) Capital accounts based on notional asset valuations.

While such voluntary reporting might be useful to certain usergroups it must of course be mentioned that the production of these reports will cost money. Moreover, if it was desired to produce such reports in a highly readable form with the use of diagrams etc. the cost could prove substantial.

5.9   Annual Review Procedures

Following parliamentary critisism of the Government's control of the NHS, the Secretary of State introduced a new set of procedures in 1982. These annual review procedures, which have been grafted on to the planning system, are formalised in nature and are designed to improve the accountability of the NHS to the Secretary of State.

The annual review procedure is a two stage process based on face-to-face discussions and comprise:

(a) An annual meeting between a Health Minister and each RHA Chairman and the Regional Team of Officers in turn;
(b) An annual meeting between an RHA Chairman and each DHA Chairman and the DMT in turn.

Clearly, the precise agenda of these meetings will vary considerably but the main topics of discussion can be summarised under two headings:

(a) Progress made in implementing developments
(b) Progress made in making better use of existing resources.

The main information base of these annual review procedures are the nationally produced performance indicators which are discussed further below.

5.10   Performance Indicators (PIs)

Performance Indicators were first published in 1983 and are seen as one of the major inputs to the annual review process. A range of PIs were produced for every DHA in England, and in some cases for every hospital. This information was distributed to every DHA and it is also publicly available.

PIs can be grouped together in five categories:

(a) Clinical Activity Measures – in this group are shown a range of measures of clinical activity such as: patient through put and average length of stay.
(b) Financial Indicators – this group contains what is essentially a range of unit cost measures. This group of PIs differs from the others in that information is produced for each individual hospital. Another interesting feature of this group is the inclusion of an expected cost per case figure derived from regression studies. This expected cost can then be compared with the actual cost per case for the hospital.
(c) Manpower Indicators – includes a range of indicators on the breakdown and utilisation of staff in the health authority.
(d) Estate Management Indicators – this group contains those indicators relating to the works function of the NHS. Thus it would include information on maintenance and energy.
(e) Miscellaneous Indicators – any other available measures not included in the above groups.

Since their publication, there has been much criticism of PIs from a number of quarters. Although some of this criticism is valid we suggest that much of it is misdirected and is based on an over estimation of what PIs can actually achieve. PIs were never intended to provide answers to questions about the performance of health authorities. Their primary use is to ask questions about performance and to identify areas where further investigation is required. For example, differences in unit costs between two DHAs do not say anything definitive about the efficiency of those DHAs. What they do is identify an area where further investigation is required either to justify the cost difference or to eliminate it. Unfortunately, we must make the point that PIs are sometimes used politically – a purpose for which they are not well suited. Turning to specific criticisms of PIs, we would make the following comments:-

(a) Coarseness – it is claimed that PIs are too coarse in nature to be of any use for local management purposes. While this is undoubtedly true, it can be replied that where PIs do not meet this aim it is for DMTs to develop their own range of PIs for local purposes and indeed a number are already doing this.

(b) Inaccuracy – PIs are criticised for being inaccurate. Again while this may be true we would point out that PIs are compiled from an information base provided by DHAs themselves. Thus any criticisms about accuracy must eventually reflect on the DHAs themselves.

It is to be hoped that the Korner developments will, in the longer term, result in improved accuracy of information collection and hence improved PIs.

(c) Lateness – it is argued that the PIs produced were produced far too late after the end of the year to be of any use. While a 12-18 month delay does seem rather excessive, it is important to realise that these were the first PIs ever produced and consequently there must be a learning effect for those involved. It is to be hoped that future sets of PIs would be produced more quickly. However, the speed of production will always be limited by the sophistication of the data collection and analysis sytems operating in DHAs. One way to improve availability is to issue estimated PIs and then compare these with actual performance. This would be compatible with the principles of standard costing.

At the time of writing, it is not clear to us what is the future of PIs. We believe that if some of the more obvious faults, such as lateness, can be ironed out then they have an important role in the accountability process.

5.11   External Audit of the NHS

In most organisations today, audit is regarded as an indispensable tool of financial control. The NHS is no exception and in fact there are two kinds of auditors external to the NHS. They can both simultaneously investigate the activities of health authorities and are:

(a) Audit staff of the DHSS audit service
(b) Audit staff of the Comptroller and Auditor General.

5.12   Audit Staff of the DHSS

The NHS Act 1948 and subsequent acts provide for the Secretary of State to appoint auditors to audit the accounts of health authorities. In reality an audit service has been established within the DHSS itself and these auditors are responsible for conducting the external audit of health authorities. On completion of their tasks, the DHSS auditors will produce a report for the health authority and the Secretary of State.

With regard to the DHSS audit, we wish to comment on two aspects of its work; its objectives and its independence.

a. Audit Objectives

The traditional role of auditors tended to be that of prevention and detection of fraud but changes in the nature of financial control and accountability have reduced the importance of this objective, and modern auditors tend to have several objectives. These can be grouped into three levels:-

i. Financial and Compliance. The auditor attempts to satisfy himself that the financial operations of the authority are properly conducted and that its financial statements are fairly presented.

ii. Efficiency. The auditor attempts to assess if the authority is conducting its activities in an economic and efficient manner and to detect the cause of any inefficiencies.

iii. Effectiveness. The auditor attempts to measure the progress made by the authority in meeting its predetermined goals.

Broadly speaking, the declared objectives of the DHSS audit service fall in line with this classification. Recent work by DHSS auditors has given greater emphasis to efficiency and effectiveness than in previous years.

The primary task of the external auditor will be that of financial compliance audit. This will involve not only an examination of the published and unpublished financial statements, but a thorough examination of the strengths and weaknesses of the financial systems which underly those statements. Only when these tasks have been performed can the external auditor consider the other aspects of efficiency audit and effectiveness audit and, even then, given his relatively limited time and limited organisational knowlegde, it is unlikely that the external auditor can make much progress in these areas. The taks of effectiveness audit and efficiency audit are more likely to be given greater emphasis by the internal auditor and this is discussed further in Chapter 8.

b.   Audit Independence

When the users of accounting information consider the report of the external auditor, it seems likely that his views on the activities of the organisation and the correctness of its financial accounts and statements will be given more credence if the auditor is perceived to be independent of the organisation. This is not a black and white question of independence or no independence, for there are various shades of grey in between. All we would say, however, is that the greater the degree of perceived independence of the auditor, the greater will be the reliance placed upon his audit report.

In the case of the limited company, the external auditor is usually perceived as being independent of the company itself, although, in reality he may be quite dependent on the company for his audit fee. With the DHSS audit service, it could be argued that the auditors are quite independent of the health authorities they audit, in that they cannot be dismissed by a health authority which takes umbrage at their report. Furthermore, they are not paid by health authorities for the work they perform. In spite of this, there is still a feeling that DHSS auditors may not be truly independent. They are sometimes regarded as internal to the larger NHS, inclusive of the DHSS, and not as an external auditor. Furthermore, there is always the possibility that their audit reports could be modified by the Secretary of State if any of the content was felt to be politically embarrassing. Consequently, there must still remain a question mark over the perceived independence of DHSS audit. On this point we should note that there have been limited moves to have some health authority accounts audited by private audit firms. However, we understand this is partly due to the need to reduce the costs of auditing certain rural health authorities, in addition to the need to break the monopoly of DHSS audit.

5.13   Audit Staff of the Comptroller and Auditor General (C & AG)

The C & AG has the statutory role of auditing all the accounts of Government departments and a wide range of other accounts of publicly financed bodies on behalf of Parliament. Consequently the C & AG has the responsibility of satisfying himself of the adequacy of systems of financial control operating in the NHS and ultimately he will be responsible for certifying the correctness of the consolidated health service accounts which are laid before Parliament. In pursuing this task, the C & AG will not be able to devote much time to detailed checking of the systems of financial control operating in individual authorities. He must rely to a great extent on the detailed work of the DHSS auditor, in the same way as the DHSS auditor will rely on the work of the internal auditor. Therefore it is necessary for him to satisfy himself as to the competence of DHSS auditors and the correctness of their work and approach.

NHS personnel are more likely to come into contact with audit staff of the C & AG when the latter are pursuing a 'value for money' type audit. The C & AG conducts such investigations, on behalf of the Public Accounts Committee, into the economy and efficiency of departmental activities and periodically health service matters will be focused upon. As an example, he undertook an investigation into the acquisition of NHS computer systems and the development of standard systems.

In conclusion, we should mention that the whole future of Government auditing is in a state of flux. Suggestions are being made that the responsibility for NHS audit be given to an expanded Audit Commission. A consequence of this may be that greater use is made of private audit firms. In our opinion these developments would lead to greater uniformity in audit standards across the public sector.

6

Allocating Resources to District Health Authorities

6.1 Two Major Questions

In Chapter 3 we discussed in some depth how money is distributed between RHAs. In this chapter we complete the resource allocation picture by considering how the RHA distributed funds between its DHAs. As mentioned in Chapter 3, there are basically three types of allocations; revenue allocations, capital allocations and earmarked allocations. We shall consider each of these separately. Throughout this chapter we continually refer to the allocations to DHAs. It is important to remember that this is an intentional oversimplification. In reality, the RHA will also allocate resources to its own services such as the blood transfusion service, the metropolitan ambulance service and RHA administration. However, this direct RHA expenditure requires only a small proportion of the funds available to the RHA, so we have restricted our attention to the allocations to DHAs.

Taking revenue allocations first, RHAs are responsible for allocating revenue monies to DHAs. We now turn to this secondary aspect of the revenue allocation process, which, in many ways, is comparable to the interregional allocation process undertaken by the DHSS. The starting point is for the RHA to be provided with the answer to two questions:

(a) *How much money is available for distribution to the DHAs?*
(b) *How should it be distributed between them?*

These questions will be considered in turn.

6.2 How Much Money is Available?

Early in each calender year, every Regional Treasurer receives a letter from the DHSS setting out the RHA's revenue allocation for the next financial year, beginning on the 1st April. This allocation is the RHA's cash limit for the daily running expenses of the health services in the region, and reflects the Government's policies on matters such as:

(a) the extent to which it will finance the impact of the current year's inflation
(b) the amount to be added for the effect of forecast inflation during the next financial year and
(c) the distribution of the development addition, which represents the amount of real growth in the DHA's revenue spending.

Some of these components of the cash limit can have compensating effects. For example, the development addition increases the money available, while the adjustment for inflation may be less than the amount required, effectively reducing the money available in real terms.

Before RHAs can formulate their policies for allocating revenue monies to the DHAs, they must be aware of the structure and the complexities of the RHA's cash limit. Similarly, all professionals in the NHS should also have an understanding of the cash limit methodology in order to appreciate the basis of the RHA's financial policy. We believe that a great deal of the criticism directed at the NHS, both internally and externally, arises from a general misunderstanding of the financial state of, and constraints imposed on, the NHS. By removing this misunderstanding, it should be possible to improve the quality of the criticism, and hopefully reduce the unconstructive content.

The question of how much money is available can be answered after considering the following four issues:

(a) the start figures
(b) the addition for forecast inflation
(c) dealing with shortfalls in inflation additions
(d) the development addition or reduction.

6.3   The Start Figures

Two recurring start figures are given to the Regional Treasurer. The first is based on the pay and price levels of the previous financial year, while the second is at the pay and price levels of the current financial year. The difference between these start figures is a combination of a number of factors such as:

(a) an allowance to cover pay and price increases in the current year
(b) the development addition or reduction for the current year.

The second start figure is in fact the recurring cash limit for the current financial year.

This second start figure becomes, in turn, the starting point of the cash limit for the following financial year. This process is illustrated in Figure 6 using the period 1982/83 to 1984/85 as an example.

The major difference between the two start figures is, of course, the adjustment for pay and price increases. This adjustment is of great significance as it reflects the extent to which the Government will finance the effect of any pay and price increases that have occurred during the current year. While it is possible that the amount provided will fully cover the effects of such inflation it seems more likely that the amount provided will be greater or less than that required. In order to identify any potential financial problem it is important to establish the adequacy of the inflation addition and this can be readily done by comparing the adjustments with the cost of pay awards for the various types of NHS staff and price increases shown in the Health Services Prices Index (HSPI).

Figure 6 – Build Up of a Revenue Cash Limit

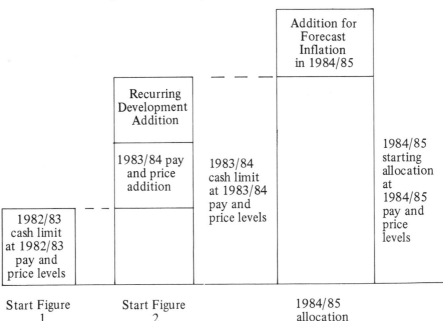

This adjustment provides the Government with a powerful financial weapon which can be used to enforce a policy of reducing public spending. If the difference between the two start figures does not fully reflect the actual cost of inflation over the twelve month period, then DHAs will be faced with a shortage of cash for their existing levels of service and might be induced to cut their present services or to use their growth addition to maintain the levels of present services. The power of the inflation adjustment lies in its shroud of financial mystique. It attracts little public attention and hostility and is therefore easy to implement. Such a use of the cash limits system has significant repercussions for each RHA and DHA. If the additions to the RHA's start figure do not reflect the actual level of inflation, they must carefully consider what action should be taken to deal with the problem. Some of the major options are considered later in this chapter.

6.4   The Addition for Forecast Inflation

From Figure 6 it can be seen that the starting point for the 1984/85 cash limit is in fact the final recurring cash limit for 1983/84. The next stage in the process is to provide a sum of money to finance the expected inflation that will occur during 1984/85. We have referred to this as the addition for forecast inflation. At the time the 1984/85 cash limit is being compiled, this figure must of course be only an estimate as the actual inflation rates are not yet known.

In dealing with this item, RHAs are faced with similar issues to that involved in the allowance for inflation in the current financial year. As an example, 1984/85 will see the operation of the pay review body for nurses and it is considered by some that the recommended pay award will be in excess of the 1984/85 cash limit addition for pay awards. At the time of allocating revenue to DHAs the RHA is unable to take actual account of any such potential hidden cuts in cash limits and thus has little option other than to pass the problem on to the DHAs. The alternative of holding a temporary regional reserve may seem superficially attractive and more certain but often results in cash being temporarily syphoned out of the system, especially when any potential underfunding may not materialise. This is discussed further in Section 6.5.

6.5   Dealing with Shortfalls in Inflation Additions

Any actual shortfalls on the inflation adjustments for the current year, together with anticipated shortfalls for the effect of forecast inflation present the RHA with two options. First, the RHA could make good the shortfall by transferring cash either from other components of the cash limit, such as the development addition, or from other allocations, such as capital. Second, the RHA could pass on the shortfall to DHAs. These two options have important implications for the management of health services by DHAs.

The first main option, where the RHA makes-good the shortfall, has the effect that cuts in the DHA's cash limits, due to the inadequate inflation provision, are avoided. This raises a constitutional, political and moral point; *should RHAs distort Government's policy to such a degree of negating the planned effects of the cash limits?* A justification for doing so lies in the financial flexibility given to RHAs by the Secretary of State, who permits limited transfers between allocations.

Transfers from capital to revenue allocations can be up to 10% of the RHA's capital allocation and if a larger transfer would be preferred, the Secretary of State will consider such a proposal. This flexibility granted by the Secretary of State recognises that RHAs may negate the effect of a cash limit squeeze on its revenue allocation. However, such a policy can only be at the expense of other types of spending, and in the case of transfers from capital, the effect would be a reduction in the capital spending of the region.

The use of transfers from capital to make good the shortfall has limited application for the RHA. Capital allocations are non-recurring and in practice they may vary enormously between years. Non-recurring monies may not be received in future years and sound financial principles dictate that the general use of non-recurring monies for recurring purposes is not to be recommended. If they are used for recurring purposes, such as to make up the recurring shortfall, they will be required beyond the current year, when their availability cannot be guaranteed. Generally, it is not advisable to use a transfer from capital to make good a recurring inflation shortfall. An exception to this rule may be perhaps for one year, when the capital transfer can subsequently be replaced by expected recurring monies. A note of caution for such short-term expediency is necessary, because future recurring additions anticipated in advance may not materialise, especially in times of economic decline and financial stringency.

Financial principles suggest that the more appropriate method of financing a recurring shortfall would be to use the development addition. Part or all of the development addition could be used to make good any shortfall on the inflation addition. One implication of such a policy is immediately obvious: the amount available for distribution to DHAs to alleviate deprivation or to finance developments is diminished. However, an inadequate pay and prices component can have an effect which would oppose the Secretary of State's policy for distributing the development addition; namely that relative deprivation should be removed by bringing the poorer DHAs up to the level of the richer DHAs. An example can illustrate the point.

Suppose the 1984/85 cash limits are being considered for two DHAs. A DHA is not deprived while B DHA is deprived. For equality to be achieved let us assume that ultimately both DHAs will require the same amount of money:

Table 7 – Illustration of the Effect of Pre-empting Development Additions

	A DHA £m	B DHA £m	Both £m
Start figure	60.0	57.0	117.0
Pay and prices addition 5%	3.0	2.9	5.9
Development addition	–	3.1	3.1
Planned cash limit for 1984/85	63.0	63.0	126.0

If the pay and price addition is inadequate and should have been 7% to reflect the eventual increases in inflation then both DHAs will require an extra sum to finance the shortfall of 2%. Consequently the RHA might decide to use part of the development addition to finance this shortfall and the following picture would then emerge:

	A DHA £m	B DHA £m	Both £m
Start figure	60.0	57.0	117.0
Pay and prices addition 7%	4.2	4.0	8.2
Development addition	–	0.8	0.8
Cash limit for 1984/85	64.2	61.8	126.0

The effect of pre-empting the development addition has been that little money has been left over to eradicate deprivation in B DHA and consequently the relative position of the two DHAs is little changed from the previous year.

By conducting such a process of transferring money from the development addition to the inflation addition the RHA may be conflicting with the Secretary of State's policy for removing relative deprivation. If these national policies are considered to be sacrosanct, then RHAs may have to strike a balance between the amounts to transfer between the cash limit components in order to implement both policies to some degree. The problem is exacerbated in those RHAs which receive small development additions or have suffered a reduction such as the four Thames RHAs. The practices regarding potential inflation shortfalls where there is minimal growth can have a critical effect on DHA services.

The second main option is for the RHA to leave any shortfall to be dealt with by each DHA as it sees fit. DHAs will then be faced with four choices, namely, transferring resources from other components of their revenue cash limit, such as its development addition; improving efficiency; transferring resources from its other allocations such as capital; cutting services. The effects and implications of both types of transfers are similar to those of the RHA's transfers considered earlier. Whether the DHA transfers from the development addition or from other allocations will depend primarily on the amount of cash available in each case. For example, DHAs with larger development additions and smaller capital allocations will obviously have a different choice to those DHAs with a smaller development addition and a larger capital allocation. An important regional variation to remember is that because of the policy behind the RAWP approach RHAs have significantly different growth rates. For 1983/84 they ranged from +1.9% in East Anglia to -0.7% in North West Thames. Similarly, within regional rates of growth, DHAs may receive an even greater range of change. Similarly the scope to release resources by efficiency improvements will vary between DHAs as they will not all have the same degree of efficiency as their starting points.

Cutting services obviously has serious implications for the DHA and its community. Three steps in a prolonged series of reductions can be identified. The initial reaction is to reduce spending on non-recurring items, such as maintenance of buildings and grounds. The second step is to take a more positive approach and look for cost reducing schemes, such as energy conservation programmes and capital intensive methods of work. This cost effective mentality should aim to reduce spending without reducing the level of service. However, as time elapses, the financial returns decrease; the third step of cost savings will then depend on real recurring reductions in service, such as staffing reductions. These three broad steps result in an initial reduction in the level of service, then a levelling out and possibly an increase as saved resources become available, followed by further, deeper cuts in spending which have the most serious effects on levels of service.

The main options in dealing with a shortfall on the addition for inflation can be summarised as shown in Figure 7.

One generalisation we believe is always valid about any financial strategy for the NHS, namely that it should be explicit and comprehensive. Government policies do not usually comply with this rule. For example, although a provision is made each year for the effects of demographic drift and technological change, the basis of this calculation has never been disclosed. An explicit policy should clearly state the overall financial position, for example that total resources will expand or contract compared to demand. It should also describe the factors that will be taken into account when allocating revenue, for example that inflation

Figure 7 – Options for Dealing with Shortfalls on the Inflation Addition

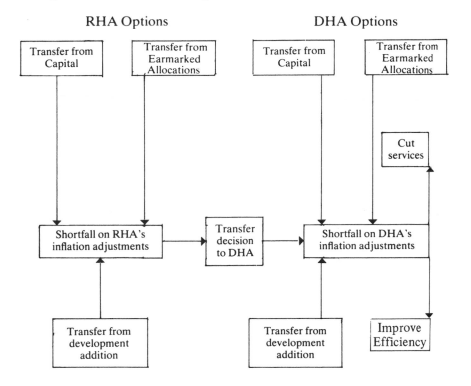

will not be financed in full and the development addition may not make up the difference, except perhaps in very deprived RHAs. This honest, revealing approach may not necessarily result in a different policy, but it will certainly improve an understanding and promote an informed debate.

Finally, it is possible that inflation additions may exceed the sums required and in this respect they can be treated as an extra development addition.

6.6   The Development Addition

The Secretary of State uses the development addition to change the position of RHAs in the RAWP target league table. RHAs can distribute the development additions between the DHAs to achieve the same goal within the region, namely equalisation between DHAs. Development additions, as their name implies, are general increases in revenue to help finance additional services. These could arise as a result of capital schemes, being the additional revenue consequences, or from a general expansion of staff, such as community nursing.

Demographic change is also an important matter to bear in mind when considering the development addition. Government's Expenditure Plans usually indicate that on average, each RHA's revenue cash limit should increase by 1% per annum so that health services could expand to cope with the growing proportion of elderly in the population. Consequently, much of the development addition of RHAs might be absorbed for this purpose and thus there might be only limited scope for using part or all of the development addition to finance any inflation shortfall. It is also clear that the smaller development additions are likely to limit the responses of some DHAs to the increasing needs of the elderly. These limitations are more severe when an inadequate development addition is considered in the context of inadequate protection against inflation. Precisely how DHAs in this financial position cope with demographic change is of great importance.

Considerable emphasis is given to the development addition and the way it is distributed between DHAs. To many people in the NHS, the whole amount of the development addition is seen as extra cash for spending on, extra staff or equipment which can contribute to an improvement in the levels of service. Very few are aware that part of the additional revenue may be required to finance existing levels of service.

6.7   How Should the Money be Distributed?

After dealing with the relatively technical aspects of the inflation adjustments to the cash limit, the RHA can direct its attention to the more public issue of distributing the development addition that remains. Two simple questions have to be answered:

(a) *How much money does each DHA have?*
(b) *How much of the RHA's allocation should each DHA have?*

The difference between these two amounts can be used to compile a league table of financial deprivation of DHAs in the region.

The answer to the first question is not difficult to provide. Details of DHA's recurring allocations are readily available from the financial information systems. These were described in Chapter 5. The amounts can be easily increased for each DHA's share of regional services or for those district costs not borne directly by the DHA. For example, most consultants' salaries can be allocated directly to the DHA which receives the benefit of their services. Other regional services, such as metropolitan ambulance services or blood transfusion services can be apportioned to DHAs with varying degrees of accuracy.

Answers to the second question are much more difficult to provide, and there may be as many different ways of answering it as there are RHAs. We have already discussed in Chapter 3 how the RAWP formula has been used to establish a measure of overall need for each RHA and to therefore calculate its target allocation. In its report, the RAWP suggested that its formula can and should be used to determine target allocations for most DHAs. A study indicated that while many problems of data inadequacy cancel out at the regional level, at the DHA level many of the assumptions, proxies, and details take on a greater significance. The RAWP method may therefore be less appropriate when allocating revenue to DHAs.

The RAWP itself recognised that its emphasis and methodology would need some adjustment to suit the circumstances of each region, and many RHAs have given some attention to these matters. Some have investigated the matter very thoroughly and consequently have refined the RAWP formula to reflect the needs of DHAs.

RHAs must, therefore, scrutinise their methods and satisfy themselves that their formulae reflect the reality of the region. If they are dissatisfied with the RAWP methodology, alternatives are available, and some are described later in this chapter. If they accept a further modified formula derived from the RAWP recommendations, then they will have a tool to determine the relative need of each DHA. They can then continue to allocate revenue to DHAs using the RAWP approach.

6.8 Allocating Revenue to DHAs

The RAWP implied that policies for revenue allocations should be based on a comparison between each DHA's actual resources and its RAWP target. Actual resources would include the:

(a) final recurring allocation for the previous year less any share of SIFT;
(b) spending by the RHA on specific services in the district;
(c) a notional share of any generally provided RHA services.

If the RHA's allocation includes a development addition, which it invariably would, the RAWP suggested that the major proportion of such a component should be allocated to those DHAs furthest away from their RAWP target allocations.

Other points that the RAWP suggested, which should be borne in mind, were: special local factors; abnormal workloads not fully reflected in costs; RCCS; ability to use additional revenue; planning considerations and the RHA's policy on reserves. To these six points, we would add a further four. These would be any shortfall on pay and price adjustments referred to earlier; the forecast targets for future years; the volatility of targets between years and the effect of demographic change. These further considerations indicate clearly that the allocation of the development addition cannot be based on a mechanical interpretation of a revenue deprivation league table. We consider each of these factors in turn:

(a) A special local factor suggested by the RAWP was the extent to which alternative facilities relieve or increase pressure on the NHS. These could include the support provided by the social services committee of the local authority because where this is limited the DHA may have to provide additional services. This could apply in particular to services for the mentally and physically handicapped and the elderly. Another example would be the level of service provided by GPs in the district. Where the population of a district has an inadequate number of GPs available, the DHA may have to provide a relatively high level of service to compensate. This may be particularly noticeable in the primary care service and the accident and emergency cover.

(b) Abnormal workloads are important to bear in mind because the effect may not be fully reflected in the estimated costs used in the formula. RAWP was not explicit on this point but we have assumed that it should reflect the cost of a service provided by the DHA which is higher than the average, because the service has to deal with a greater number of patients and achieves a higher throughput.

(c) The RCCS are important to take into account when RHAs are changing to a RAWP approach. Many DHAs will have an RCCS commitment arising from decisions taken outside the RAWP procedures, and finance for the RCCS would have been assumed at an appropriate level. The RAWP approach could leave some DHAs with commitments of RCCS that exceed its development addition. The RAWP advocated an approach which recognises these difficulties. We have inferred that a phased introduction of the RAWP approach was not only preferred but essential on financial grounds.

Referring to later RAWP comments on planning considerations it seems to us that the RAWP also implied a balance between a general development addition and an addition for RCCS. This may be particularly important in some DHAs which are relatively small and may find any RCCS a relatively higher proportion of its revenue allocation and therefore a significant additional cost.

(d) The ability to absorb revenue was mentioned earlier in this chapter in regard to the availability of infrastructure and manpower. Clearly the removal of acute deprivation depends on a DHA employing more staff and providing them with the tools of their trade. Any development addition spent on other items may not remove deprivation but could merely balance the books in terms of the RAWP target league table. We believe that this aspect is important in another respect. It also governs the rate of progress towards target. By taking account of a DHAs ability to spend any extra money wisely, a RHA is implicitly fixing the rate of progress towards financial equality, and we consider it vital for RHAs to have regard to a timescale for the implementation of this policy. Rather than consider the ability of DHAs to respond to extra money in the forthcoming year, it seems more constructive to look ahead and assess how long it is likely to take the deprived DHAs to appoint staff and provide the infrastructure it needs. The length of the period may have important consequences. For example, if it will take twenty years for the relevant staff to be available for all the deprived DHAs in a region, the RHA and the DHAs will have to tolerate deprivation for that period. Such a proposition may be unacceptable to many authorities. To recognise deprivation and be unable to remove it for such a long period may arouse feelings of futility and desperation. In such circumstances an alternative may have to be found. This could include an expansion of contractual arrangements, in line with a policy of greater co-operation with the private health services. Alternatively, a rearrangement of cross boundary flows may prove useful so that the near target DHAs provide a greater service to their poorer neighbours. As this may often be to the detriment of the resident population, such a policy may be regarded as equalising misery, and is contrary to the policy of levelling-up resources.

A plea often heard from DMTs was that deprivation could be overcome by greater district self-sufficiency. While the RAWP recognised that district self-sufficiency was not the aim of its formula, progress towards equal access to health services for people at equal risk may only be possible by pursuing a policy of moving towards greater self-sufficiency but not necessarily complete self-sufficiency. If additional resources for a DHA are used to reduce deprivation they must be deployed in a mixture of three ways:

(i) the DHA could provide health care for those residents already travelling to a neighbouring district for treatment;

(ii)   it could provide health care for those residents not receiving any of the treatment needed;

(iii) it could provide health care for the population of neighbouring districts.

In all three cases, an expansion in the services provided is required to reduce deprivation in real terms, which implies a policy of greater self-sufficiency. Merely increasing DHA's revenue allocations without a complementary policy for the redeployment or expansion of real resources will only result in equality of financial resources and not of the health services resources. We recognise, however, that given the probable low rates of growth in NHS funds it will take a long time to achieve such an improvement in services.

(e) This leads up to the fifth matter considered by the RAWP namely planning considerations. Suffice to say that the NHS Planning System has proved complex and cumbersome to operate, but in our view, such a mechanism, is indispensable. The RAWP outlined some of the main features of planning as developing priority services; closures; changes of use; patterns of delivery of care and centres of excellence. Clearly, as we have already indicated in relation to self-sufficiency, the allocation of money must be in harmony with a planned contraction and expansion of health services in each of the districts. However, it is important to be pragmatic. Precise information on the effects of these priorities is unlikely to be readily available, if at all, and we cannot avoid the conclusion that the balance between financial allocations and service changes is more a matter of judgement rather than fact.

Theoretically, the problem should not arise in the long term. If the RAWP formula reflects the need for resources, then the planning system should point out those same needs and provide some means of fulfilment. Thus finance would match changes in service. Such precision is unlikely because the two processes draw from different data. As the RAWP formula often uses proxies and notional adjustments it could produce an answer quite unrelated to the planning systems view of deprivation. The swings and roundabouts effect is unlikely to operate. This emphasises the need for cohesion and a balance between the two sets of information.

(f) The need to hold financial reserves is an important aspect of any organisation's financial policy. The RAWP recommended that these should be kept to a minimum in order to secure the most equitable distribution possible and should be concentrated wherever possible at the DHA. Our interpretation of minimum is derived from the distinction between caution and contingency. In times of unpredictable inflation and limited growth, a RHA may hold substantial reserves in order to protect DHAs from the realities of financial life. Such reserves may not be used to improve the service and as DHAs are responsible public bodies, such choices between caution and contingency would be better left to them. The need for contingency reserves will always exist. Unusual or unpredictable occurrences, such as an unexpected large loss to be written off, arise from time to time, and the RHA can use its contingency reserve as an insurance policy.

Specific reserves are often used for particular service developments such as the RCCS and the revenue consequences of medical appointments (RCMA). When some RHAs approve developments, such as the appointment of a consultant, they have often made a specific allocation to finance the revenue consequences. If the appointment is delayed, then finance must be reserved or earmarked until the time that it is required. Invariable, delays in implementing these specific service developments arise. This phenomenon of slippage, which seems to bedevil almost every organisation's programme, can result in a considerable amount of money being accumulated in specific reserves.

(g) Shortfalls on pay and price additions were not mentioned by the RAWP as a factor to take into account when allocating development additions. This matter was dealt with earlier in this chapter. It is sufficient to note here that if the RHA prefers a policy of levelling-up, then it must look at the effect of the whole allocation, and not just the development addition. It is the 'comprehensive' part of the 'explicit and comprehensive' financial policy referred to earlier.

(h) Forecast targets are of major importance when considering the RAWP target league tables. It is shortsighted to change the financial state of a DHA in the short term and then have to reverse or significantly alter the position in a few years' time. Two examples illustrate the point well. First, suppose a DHA is considerably under its RAWP target and is an obvious candidate for revenue growth. Also consider that the DHA will be opening a large DGH in four years' time and the additional revenue funds received for the running of that hospital will raise the DHA up to its target. During the intervening period, if the RHA was to assign growth monies to the DHA as part of its policy of equalisation then this could cause problems when the DGH eventually opened. These growth monies might have been committed by the DHA in various ways so that when the DGH was opened, sufficient finance may not be available to utilise it completely as the revenue was being used elsewhere. Perhaps an appropriate policy for the use of growth monies would be either to make small additions each year on the explicit understanding that the DHA will husband them carefully so that they can eventually be used to finance the RCCS of the DGH. Alternatively, the RHA could withhold development additions until the RCCS had to be financed, then large appropriate development additions could be provided. The effect of the alternatives over the long term would be the same.

The second example of the need for a look ahead is where the DHA is near to target but a large increase in its population is forecast causing an increased need for resources. This effect may be found in those DHAs with new town developments. In these cases it is not very sensible to freeze or reduce the DHAs' revenue allocation just because it is near to target now, and then to suddenly inject relatively large development additions as the additional population arrives. It seems to be more sensible if the DHA is allocated development additions which enable it to be prepared for the additional population rather than have to respond to it. Again as with the first example, the comparison of the DHA's target with its allocation, in the long term, would produce the same result if resources were allocated by either method.

(i)   RAWP targets for DHAs may prove to be very volatile as a result of changes in the base data of the formula. For example, small population shifts in a small DHA could result in relatively large changes in the DHA's RAWP target. Similarly, changes in mortality rates from one year to the next could radically affect the target. Clearly the RHA cannot have a sensible approach to resource allocation when DHA targets are constantly changing. A DHA might be below target one year and the RHA might boost its allocation to bring it closer to target. Subsequently small changes to the base data of the DHA might reduce its RAWP target and place it in the position of being above target in the following year. The RHA can hardly take away the money it has just given. One way round this problem would be to stabilise DHA targets over a period of years by fixing the base data for that period. For example, mortaility rates could be held constant for say three years and then reviewed and changed as necessary. A note of caution is still required with this approach, as even with the three-yearly review, it is still possible to pick an unrepresentative year for a DHA. Its three-year target will be fixed at an inappropriate level and when reviewed again, may result in a sudden change. Such statistical expediences must therefore be implemented with great care and caution.

Volatile revenue targets have been experienced with some DHAs. For example, the distance from revenue target of one district known to us changed, over a year, from 15% under target to 4% under target as a result of a changed target. Such considerable swings were ironed out of some RHAs RAWP league tables by banding DHAs. The bandings used were related to the extent to which the DHAs were over- or under-target. Some examples of bandings could be 'above target', 'slightly deprived', 'deprived',or 'very deprived'. The banding approach is likely to prove indispensible in achieving a reasonable degree of consistency between years.

(j) The final matter to take account of in making allocations to DHAs is demographic change. We have already referred to the need for NHS resources to grow by about 1% per annum to provide for demographic changes. The amounts required by individual DHAs may well range around this figure. For example, DHAs with new towns which conventionally have young populations, are likely to have a slower growth in the proportion of its elderly than a DHA with inner city areas, where the younger population is migrating. Where such a DHA is close to target it may be a narrow view for the RHA to ignore the demographic indicators and adhere rigidly to the RAWP methodology.

These ten factors outlined cannot be combined in any precise or mechanical way. Circumstances vary between RHAs and the various factors will assume differing degrees of significance in different regions. The only rule that can be consistently applied is that the weight to give to each factor is a matter of the RHA's judgement. That judgement can be improved by an understanding of the financial profile of the NHS and the region.

6.9 The RAWP Approach in Practice

A recent study conducted by the National Association of Health Authorities (NAHA) has thrown some light on the way in which RHAs actually apply the RAWP approach sub-regionally. The study involved issuing questionnaires to all the RHAs in England and summarising the responses obtained.

The study indicated that all RHAs bar one use the RAWP methodology for sub-regional allocations but all have found it necessary to modify the national RAWP methodology. Some of the modifications made are listed here:

(a) Mental Illness and Mental Handicap Services – None of the RHAs

use the RAWP methodology for these services and different approaches to resource allocations are used in each RHA.
(b) Regional Specialties – In many RHAs, designated regional specialties
     are taken out of the RAWP process altogether and are separately
     protected.
(c) Deprivation Factors – Some RHAs have introduced an additional
     factor into the RAWP formula to take account of relative deprivation
     between DHAs.

All RHAs in the country reported that the distribution of any development addition is based on the distance a DHA is from its RAWP target.
However, this process is somewhat mitigated by the fact that most RHAs
still make some provision for RCCS. This RCCS element is bound to pre-
empt some of the funds in the development addition.

One point of criticism that must be noted is that most RHAs reported
that they did not employ any mechanism to reconcile the RAWP target
setting process with the process of service planning in the short term and
the long term. This absence of a link between planning and resource
allocation strikes one as illogical.

6.10   Alternatives to the RAWP Method

As we have already mentioned, the RAWP formula may need considerable refinement before it can be used to calculate DHA revenue targets.
These adjustments may be so extensive that RHAs can reasonably ask
themselves whether an alternative to RAWP would be more appropriate.
Three main methods are discussed here which deserve careful consideration, one is capital led allocations; the second is allocations derived from
annual programmes and hence strategic plans, while the third is a
method employed in the USA namely that of diagnostic related groups.

a. Capital Led Revenue Allocations

The implicit assumption in this method is that deprivation in a DHA can be
overcome by the injection of capital. The additional infrastructure ultimately provided will generate additional revenue spending thus reflecting an
increase in the level of service in the district. In outline, the process would
begin by identifying the need for capital investment, followed by the implementation of the capital scheme, then a subsequent increase in the DHA's
revenue allocation to finance the associated revenue consequences.

An advantage of such an approach to revenue allocation arises as a result of the generally limited financial flexibility of DHAs which may have some difficulty in financing large RCCS from general development additions which may have been spread thinly around the region. A policy of diverting money to those DHAs requiring RCCS funds may be the only financially viable strategy available to some RHAs. Adopting such an approach ony complies with our criteria 'explicit and comprehensive' refered to earlier if it is recognised that deprivation is being partly overcome by capital investment.

Three major weaknesses of this approach are:

(a) no reliable information is available on the type of capital investment needed to overcome deprivation;
(b) capital investment overcomes only certain types of deprivation, usually related to the provision of hospital care;
(c) how does a RHA deal with a DHA which is relatively well provided with capital but relatively deprived of revenue?

Indicators of capital deprivation are usually comprised of a target stock value or quantity compared to the actual stock level. No information is provided about the type of deficiencies or relative over-provision. With this approach it is assumed that any type of capital will remove the deprivation, but if it is of an inappropriate type, such as doubling the size of an already adequate DGH, the level of health services will not develop in the required sectors. For this method of allocation to be effective, it must be linked to some overall strategy of programmed capital investment. This information can be derived from the regions' strategic and operational plans.

A further difficulty of this method is that it only deals with capital deprivation. Manpower deprivation such as shortages of community staffing or specialist clinicians would not be reflected in this approach. The need for such developments would be established by the strategic and operational planning process, and it may be possible to expand the capital led revenue allocation process to include such factors.

It can be seen that the two major objections to capital led revenue allocations can be overcome by using the region's planning system. This process may in itself provide the basis for revenue allocations, and we now turn to assess this possibility.

b. *Revenue Allocations Derived from Annual Programmes*

DHAs are responsible for planning and are therefore required to participate in the NHS planning process. It is worth noting here that annual programmes are the expression of the implementation of the first two years of the ten year strategic plan. Any corporate plan is based on an assessment of the needs of the community and indicates how these needs will be met. The DHA's strategy should be no exception and this gives us the key. If DHAs are required to identify need in order to prepare its ten-year strategy, and produce an annual programme to state how that need will be met over the next two years, this programme can be used as the basis of the RHA's revenue allocation mechanism.

The principle would be that within its resources the RHA would provide the finance required to implement the operational plan. This method would be financially viable. Precise, earmarked financing would not be involved, as the simplest and most flexible method would be for the allocation of the development addition to reflect the plans in broad terms.

The greatest advantage of this method is that it combines allocation with planning and two main benefits of this link are that planning becomes more realistic and also more meaningful. Realism is attained by firstly building a financial base into the planning process and secondly recognising the financial requirements of the implementation of the plans. Planning becomes more effective because it becomes the means for attracting resources. The financial incentive to plan is the ideal catalyst to improve the quality and regularity of planning in the NHS.

A drawback of this approach is the lack of objectivity. It seems to us that a measure of need for planning purposes is imbued with subjectivity. Measures of need may differ between DHAs and it may be difficult to reach agreement on relative need. To overcome this difficulty, it is important that the RHA establishes its planning methodology to ensure comparability and if objectivity cannot be attained at least the subjectivity can be dealt with openly. Such openness may produce an understanding that can be generally accepted as reflecting relative need between DHAs.

c. Diagnostic Related Groups

Diagnostic Related Groups (DRG) are a concept originally developed in the USA but which has recently been creating interest in Great Britain as having applicability to resource allocation. Let us first describe what DRGs are then discuss their potential for use in resource allocation in the NHS.

DRGs are a complex scheme for classifying hospital in-patients into a number of groups such that each group contains patients who have diagnostically related conditions. Four guidelines are set down for the construction of DRGs:

(a) the groups formulated must be medically meaningful

(b) the groups must be based on readily available data
(c) there must be a managable number of groups which must, in turn, be mutually exclusive and exhaustive. A figure of less than 500 DRGs is suggested as a guideline.
(d) each group must have a statistically stable distribution of length of stay and cost. Failure to achieve this would mean that DRGs would have little use for resource allocation purposes.

Once DRGs have been formulated it then becomes possible to classify all hospital in-patients into one of these groups. This then provides the basis for a method of resource allocation. Hospitals could be funded on the following basis:-

Funds available = Planned number of patients in each DRG
X Budgeted cost per patient for each DRG

Thus the allocation of funds to a hospital would be arrived at by combining the estimated number of patients and the budgeted cost per patient for each DRG and summating for all DRGs. This is in fact the method employed by the United States Federal Government to fund the Medicare Programme. In the first year of the programme, the hospitals will only receive 25% of their costs funded through DRGs but over a four year period it is intended to move to full funding through DRGs.

Although DRGs may have considerable merit as a tool of planning or performance review, we cannot believe they would have much applicability to resource allocation from RHAs to DHAs within the present financing structure of the NHS. There would appear to be several major obstacles to their use and some of these are discussed below:

(i)   DRGs only deal with hospital in-patients and do not cover hospital out-patients or community services. Thus there would be a major limitation in using DRGs to allocate resources to DHAs especially in a service where community care is being emphasised.
(ii) Information systems in the NHS are insufficiently advanced to be able to cope with a system of DRGs. This would be especially true in the field of costing systems. The Korner Working Party F proposals on specialty costing would not meet the needs of a DRG costing system and the costs of treating patients in each DRG are an essential component. Again, it seems to us that only the development of patient costing systems would fully meet this need.
(iii) The biggest problem with the DRG approach concerns the fact that health authorities are cash limited. Using a DRG approach to resource

allocation could result in a situation where the total funds required by a DHA is greater than that which the RHA is able or prepared to give. For better or for worse the funding of the NHS is based on a top-down rationing process whereby a nationally determined sum is shared out between the constituent health authorities on some equitable basis. On the other hand, the DRG approach represents a bottom-up standards process whereby the resources required by a DHA are computed by reference to the number of patients requiring treatment and the costs of providing that treatment. The problem of course is that the resources required by DHAs would probably be greater than that which the Government is prepared to provide.

From what has been said above, it can be seen that we have considerable doubts about the use of DRGs as a method of allocating resources to DHAs. However, it seems possible that the DRG approach might have greater applicability within the DHA in allocating resources to individual units.

Unfortunately, we believe that the use of such a method within the DHA might result in the hospital based services monopolising resources to a degree greater than at present. Using DRGs to allocate resources to units might well result in a situation where community services get what is left over after the hospitals have had their share. This in itself would reverse the trend towards a greater emphasis on community care.

6.11   Combination of Methods

We have now described four different approaches to the allocation of revenue monies to DHAs, namely:

(a) the RAWP approach
(b) capital led revenue allocations
(c) revenue allocations derived from annual programmes
(d) DRG costing.

It is important to realise, however, that these four methods are not mutually exclusive. It is not a case of using one method and ignoring the others; they can be used in combinations. For example, the RHA could set aside funds for the 'cinderella' services for geriatrics and mentally handicapped. These funds could be distributed between DHAs to enable them to finance their annual programmes for these services. The rest of the RHA's funds intended for the acute and general care group could then be distributed among the DHAs according to RAWP principles. Similarly, part of the regional development addition could be used to finance the

RCCS, leaving a balance to be allocated by using the RAWP principles.

6.12   Selecting a Method of Revenue Allocation

It is clearly the RHAs' responsibility to devise an appropriate method of allocating revenue to DHAs and regionally provided services. The criteria that we would suggest to RHAs in their search are first, the method must be sensitive to the regional circumstances; second it must be based on a generally acceptable measurement of need; third, it must be made explicit to DHAs and fourth, it must comprehensively embrace all the components' of the revenue cash limit.

Our assessment is that revenue allocations based on annual programmes will probably be the most appropriate method in most regions. It would fit all the criteria above and in particular, because it would be based on regionally provided information, it would be particularly sensitive to the DHAs' requirements. This aspect is critical in the NHS which is comprised of some relatively small DHAs which in many cases may not be able to cope with substantial, increased demands on their finances. Furthermore it would substantially overcome the criticism made in 6.9 about the lack of reconciliation between planning and resource allocation.

6.13   Allocating Capital to DHAs

There are three main types of capital expenditure:

(a) minor capital
(b) major capital
(c) RHA capital.

Major capital expenditure is incurred directly by RHAs, and its allocation to specific schemes should be determined by the operation of the 'NHS Planning System'. Consequently, it is not considered in this section. Similarly, RHA capital is required for items of spending such as regional computing facilities, expensive medical equipment and a regional land programme. While regional variations can be numerous, the schemes financed under the heading of RHA capital should also be determined by the 'NHS Planning System'.

Minor capital is designed for small schemes and its use can be devolved entirely to DHAs. Variations on the method of allocation are probably as numerous as there are RHAs, but each has one general aim, namely to allocate each DHA an appropriate share of such capital. An appropriate technique should take into account the use that is made of the allocation and it is in this respect that the definition of small schemes is relevant.

Some RHAs define a small scheme as one costing less than £100,000. Other RHAs may use a higher limit of, say, £250,000. While such differences may require a different emphasis in distribution, the RAWP implied that its revenue weighted population could be used as the mechanism. Having decided on the amount to be allocated as minor capital, the RHA would then give DHAs a minor capital allocation in direct proportion to their revenue weighted populations. Initially, it is difficult to see why such an approach, which is designed for revenue allocations, should be helpful in respect of capital. However, it should be remembered that capital can be used for schemes which are similar in nature to some revenue schemes. In this respect, minor capital can be seen as an extension of revenue spending. Furthermore, these capital allocations can usually be transferred to revenue as required by DHAs.

An alternative to this approach is to distribute minor capital in proportion to each DHA's capital stock. In Chapter 3 we outlined how such a valuation could be completed using the RAWP methodology. Within regions, such an approach may be considered unsatisfactory, and a comprehensive review of assets may be preferred. This could be comprised of an inventory of all capital stock, including an assessment of age and condition. These valuations could then be used as the basis for future allocations of minor capital.

Thirdly, one radical method which does not seem to have been attempted is the RAWP's 'bidding approach'. While we have concluded that it may well be impractical at a national level, the proposition is more attractive for use within RHAs for one main reason: the administrative process required to produce the preferences of each DHA are relatively easy to manage at this level. DHAs could bid for various allocations of minor capital, subsequently paying the appropriate rates of interest which they are prepared to finance from their revenue allocations. The great advantage of this approach within RHAs is that each DHA can influence the amount of minor capital that it is to receive. A disadvantage is that the RHA may be placed in a position where the DHA's bids exceed the amount the RHA wishes to allocate, and therefore cannot be met. Consequently DHAs will have to respond quickly to a lower level of capital than desired and planned for. This uncertainty is not conducive to good management.

A further matter to be considered is the use of the DHA's interest payments. RHAs may be tempted to transfer this 'income' to revenue and use it to quicken the pace towards equality. DHAs may prefer the interest payments to be used to increase the amount of capital available so as to ensure that the requirements of each DHA can be met in full. Such matters can only be resolved after considering regional and district circumstances and the sums involved could be the topic of regional consultation and negotiation.

A significant matter is how the RHAs share out their total capital to each of the three types of capital, namely minor capital, major capital and RHA capital. Formulae cannot be recommended for this task. It is for the RHA to develop priorities, preferably in consultation with DHAs, which can help in deciding how much capital should be included in each category. One likelihood is almost certain: each category will require more than the amount available and a reasonable balance over a long time-scale should be the main aim.

6.14   Earmarked Allocations

The earmarked allocations to RHAs that we referred to in Chapter 3 are relatively standardised in the way they are applied to each RHA. When we look at the earmarked allocations to DHAs, the picture is much more complex. While the national earmarked allocations, such as joint finance, tend to be allocated to DHAs by using the DHSS methodology, the range of regional earmarked allocations can be as numerous as the RHAs. These regional variations are sometimes classified as top-slicing; in this section we discuss how some of these earmarked funds are distributed between DHAs.

a. RCCS

Allocations to specifically finance RCCS are still used by some RHAs. These could be for all RCCS, or just for the major RCCS, say, over £100,000 in total. The reason for continuing with such specific allocations is often related to the limited amount of development additions available to DHAs. Smaller DHAs may require relatively large amounts of additional finance to meet their RCCS, and these can exceed the total of any general development addition. In these circumstances, the use of specific RCCS allocations may be both appropriate and useful.

b. Revenue Consequences of Clinical Developments

Generally, clinical developments include new medical techniques which may require additional resources in order that they may be refined and generally available. Some RHAs allocate revenue specifically for such developments. As for RCCS, the justification for these allocations is that the RHA can provide finance to plan and encourage clinical developments.

c. RCMA

As RHAs are responsible for appointing and deploying most consultants, they may feel obliged to provide revenue to pay for the clerical support and clinical costs directly associated with a new appointment. These can be reflected in specific allocations for RCMA.

d. Revenue Costs of Regional Specialties

Some DHAs will provide specialties which are accessible to a substantial proportion of, or all of, the population in a region. An example is kidney transplants. If it can be demonstrated that such a typical cross-boundary flow is not adequately reflected in the normal revenue allocation process, such as the RAWP formula, then the RHA may top-slice its revenue allocation and finance regional specialties directly. While this method of finance tends to be associated with particular specialities, it can also be used for whole services. One example is the services for the mentally handicapped, where large institutions provide facilities for large parts of a region. If the costs cannot be adequately reflected in the RAWP formula, the services could be financed from an earmarked allocation.

   Such an approach can be defended because of the regional nature of the specialty or service. Because it is of regional importance, the RHA may feel justified in having a direct financial involvement.

e. Earmarked Capital Allocations

These earmarked allocations would tend to apply only to the capital schemes which will be financed from a DHA's minor capital allocation. For example, if the RHA wished to encourage the refurbishment of obsolete ambulance stations, it may do so by including its own metropolitan ambulance service schemes in its capital budget, and giving the appropriate DHAs an earmarked allocation for non-metropolitan ambulance services. The advantages of such an allocation process is that regional priorities can be pursued.

f. Joint Finance

The main purpose of joint finance is outlined in Chapter 3. The method of allocation within regions should correspond with the method used by the DHSS for allocating joint finance to RHAs, namely on the basis of population served. However, one difficulty arises in those local authority areas in which there are more than one DHA. In such circumstances, the allocation could be either:

(a) into a local authority pool
(b) to each DHA.

The advantage of using a local authority pool is that priorities can be assessed and balanced across the whole area covered by the social services. However, constitutionally, such monies cannot be used without the consent of the DHAs, and this factor leads us to conclude that allocations direct to DHAs would be more appropriate. In this way, DHAs can directly control the use of the allocation and ensure that the health services in their districts will benefit from the sum available.

One final matter in relation to earmarked allocations is the principle of top-slicing. It often causes great consternation among Treasurers. Some seem to be firmly in favour of it, while others are adamently opposed to it in principle. It is important to understand that while many RHAs continue to top-slice allocations, such a principle is not sacrosanct. The opposing view would be that the money should be distributed to DHAs generally, leaving them to pursue a particular development if they attached a high enough priority to it. Top-slicing can be seen as an erosion of DHA autonomy. Conversely, its abolition can be seen by RHAs as usurping their role.

7

Priorities and Planning in District Health Authorities

7.1. Corporate and Functional Planning

Earlier approaches to planning in health authorities could be described as functional, or departmental, planning. This implies that planning was a series of separate exercises performed for the various functions of the health authority. Although the individual plans might have been co-ordinated in such a way as to eliminate possible duplications of effort, functional planning could not be said to be planning for the authority as a whole. On examination, it could frequently be found that the individual plans did not support each other and quite often contradicted each other.

Corporate planning is an alternative approach which emphasises planning for the organisation as a whole. It means planning for the authority in total, rather than by department or function, and implies that planning is carried out within defined and agreed objectives. This corporate approach is the basis of the NHS Planning System and has been adopted in many health authorities. It is effected largely through planning teams for groups of services. These consider the services provided for particular classes of patients, such as the elderly or the mentally handicapped, and the result is that the services provided are planned in a comprhensive and co-ordinated way. Taking services for the elderly as an example, plans for community services would be co-ordinated with the hospital services to ensure that the effects of planned changes in one service are reflected and supported in the other. Similarly, changes in the patern of out-patient treatment at hospitals would be reflected in the plans of the ambulance service, a service which may be radically affected by the proposed changes. A more difficult area is in co-ordinating the services changes of DHAs and local authority and voluntary services. This must also be included in plans.

The advantage of the corporate approach is that the authority should be more effective in achieving its objectives. It would move forward as a whole rather than the alternative in which each function advances independently. It is in this context of corporate planning that we consider priorities and planning in DHAs.

In Chapter 4 we have already discussed in some detail the nature of the formal 'NHS Planning System' as developed by the DHSS and operated in health authorities. In our experience, staff who operate the system and are affected by it have mixed views about the usefulness of this formal planning system. Most people seem to accept that some sort of planning system is necessary if only for the purpose of assuring Parliament, which is the ultimate paymaster of the NHS, that an attempt is being made to ensure that funds are to be utilised in accord with national priorities. However, opinions differ as to the usefulness of the NHS Planning System within health authorities. Some consider it to be totally adequate for the planning needs of their authority while, at the other extreme the attitude of some staff towards the Planning System is that it is only one more requirement in the seemingly endless and unnecessary series of returns that have to be submitted to the DHSS. Consequently, in this chapter we are concerned with the need for planning and especially its financial aspects. Although we shall relate planning in general to the formal NHS Planning System, our initial aim will be to consider:

(a) why DHAs should undertake the task of planning the provision of health services;
(b) the benefits of planning for DHAs;
(c) the contents of DHA plans.

Since this chapter is mainly concerned with the role of finance in planning, the remainder deals with some of the financial and economic 'techniques' available for use in planning.

7.2   Why DHAs Need to Plan

The alternative to planning in organisations is a style of management which merely responds to immediate pressures, with the result that the organisation is likely to lurch from one crisis to another. For example, a DHA may suffer bad publicity, and may respond by pouring resources into dilapidated long-stay units, only to reverse that policy at a later date as a result of additional pressure from clinicians in the acute and general sector. Clearly, a more rational approach to change is desirable, and this is where planning assists.

Anyone who has observed planning procedures in an organisation can testify that planning is not a free good. The setting up of a planning system in a large organisation such as a DHA will be aware that planning commits the organisation to employ specialist planning staff, and requires most staff to be involved to some extent in planning procedures. In a modern context, expenditure will also be incurred on items such as computing facilities and printing of documents, and consequently, however simple the planning system, there will always be some cost involved in its operation. It therefore follows from this that if organisations undertake planning it must be for very sound reasons. Consequently, it is a simple argument that DHAs should only plan and set up planning systems if the benefits obtained are greater than the costs incurred in setting up and operating such systems. To argue for planning is therefore to elucidate and prefer the benefits that planning brings, and also to accept the costs.

While we will argue the case for planning, it is not possible to draw general conclusions about the costs and benefits of planning systems. The degree of planning undertaken by a DHA must be assessed individually on its merits. However, it is notoriously difficult to quantify the benefits of a system of planning and so the case for planning must to some degree, rest on judgement.

7.3   The Benefits of Planning

What then are these supposed benefits that will flow from a system of planning? Before answering that question we should first discuss four factors which are basic to all organisations including DHAs:

(a) organisational objectives
(b) limited resources
(c) time scale of decision-making
(d) uncertainty.

a. Organisational Objectives

Before setting out on a journey of some sort, it is necessary for the individual to know where he is at present, and where he wishes to be at on some future date. Plans for a journey cannot be formulated until the starting point of the journey and its final destination are known. Moreover, if one sets out on a journey without an adequate plan, it is more than likely that one will not reach the intended destination. Similarly with organisations, it is not possible for managers to make rational decisions about the future course of the organisation until they are aware of where the organisation is at present and where it wishes to be. Thus we have the idea of the organisational objective.

Although most if not all organisations have some sort of objective these are not always explicitly stated. Furthermore, the overall organisational objective may be further divided into a hierarchy of sub-objectives, each tier of which is more specific than the one above. In the case of a limited company, we will usually find that the organisational objective will be stated in terms of increased profitability or increased sales. This objective can then be supported by production plans, sales campaigns and profit margins.

In DHAs the absence of a profit element creates problems for identifying and quantifying an overall objective. If, for example we say that the overall objective of a DHA is to maximise the health services of the local community, this tells us nothing concrete. Perhaps the objective can therefore only be expressed in terms of a number of sub-objectives such as reduction in waiting times, reduction of child-mortality, prevention of cancer. The detailed objectives of the DHA will of course be determined in the light of its priorities. We have already argued in Chapter 4 that the priorities of a DHA will be arrived at by a process of adapting national guidelines to meet local conditions. Once the priorities have been decided, the objectives of the DHA will flow from this. For example, the DHA might decide that one priority must be reduced waiting times for ENT surgery. From this priority will flow a precise objective which quantifies the desired reduction in waiting times and a specific proposal will be produced to enable that objective to be achieved. Alternatively, a priority might be to improve the speech therapy service and from this will flow an objective showing the improvement actually required together with a proposal for achieving it. The key point is that unless the priorities of the DHA are known, decisions about objectives cannot be made rationally and consequently the organisation will only drift along.

b. Limited Resources

Organisations and individuals are confronted by the fact that the resources available to them are not infinite. Consequently, decision-making should recognise the limit of resources and must be concerned with maximising the use of limited resources. This resource constraint applies to DHAs as much as to other organisations.

What has been said gives us the key to another reason why DHAs must plan. Decisions on plans must be made in such a way that progress is made towards the DHA's pre-determined objectives while at the same time ensuring that full use is made of the limited resources that are available. One way in which this can be done is by a system of planning which will enable priorities to be assessed and ranked, and for specific proposals for developments and cuts to be considered in relation to each other. In the absence of planning, decisions will be made that may either bear no relation to the priorities and objectives of the DHA or will result in the under-utilisation of the resources available.

c. *Time Scale of Decision-Making*

It is a fact of life that some decisions take longer to come to fruition than others. For example, consider the building of a new hospital. It may take up to 15 years from the time of deciding to build the hospital to the acceptance of the first patients. If we are to ensure that the hospital is not being under-utilised we must make certain that it is ready to accept patients as soon as construction is completed. However, the running of a hospital depends on many other factors, for example, the availability of trained manpower, such as nurses, and specialist equipment. These are not always available at short notice and consequently if we are to ensure that the hospital is to be put to maximum use, we must ensure that these other resources are available when required. The only way we can do this is by a system of planning.

A similar example to this concerns the construction of a new hospital in a New Town. Ideally, construction of the hospital should begin early enough to ensure that its facilities are available when the New Town has developed to the extent that large numbers of people are resident there. If construction of the hospital commences too late, then residents may not have the access to health services they require. On the other hand if construction begins too soon, the hospital may be under-utilised for a period of time. Again this demonstrates the need for a system of planning.

d. *Uncertainty*

Unfortunately for DHAs, we live in an uncertain world. To forecast the precise state of the DHA's environment in one year's time let alone ten, may require brave assumptions. A number of factors contribute to this overall level of uncertainty, and while most people recognise the type of uncertainty that affects commercial organisations, such as uncertainty about the demand for products, or uncertainty about interest rates, not everyone recognises the uncertainty that faces DHAs.

Three main elements are:
(i)   uncertainty about future resources
(ii) uncertainty about the size and structure of the catchment populations
(iii) uncertainty about changes in medical technology.

Furthermore, the smaller the DHA the greater is the degree of uncertainty and the greater the impact on planning. As far as planning is concerned, there are two aspects of uncertainty which we need to consider:

(i)   forecasting
(ii) contingency plans.

(i)   Forecasting Many of the factors which contribute towards uncertainty are not completely unpredictable in nature, and some effort can and should be made to assess potential changes in these factors. Consider for example, a decline in the number of babies being born in a particular district. If the DHA is unaware of the possibility of such a change then it is probable that the authority would find itself with under-utilised facilities. Similarly, if there was an increase in the birth rate, the DHA could find itself unable to provide adequate maternity facilities. To some extent, it is possible to obtain projections of birth rates and DHAs can avail themselves of such information. In particular, population and demographic forecasts can be obtained from the Office of Population Censuses and Surveys. Such forecasts can provide the starting point of a careful consideration of the future.

(ii)   Contingency Plans There are many factors which are more or less unpredictable. The level of resources available in future years is a typical example, where eventual allocations of capital and revenue development additions may vary considerably from forecasts. In order that it can cope adequately with such uncertainty it is desirable that DHAs adopt a system of what is termed contingency planning. By this we mean that plans are formulated in such a way that appropriate, planned alternatives are available which can be introduced in response to unpredictable changes. The possibility of variations in resource availability should be planned for by having a series of strategic and operational plans based on different resource assumptions. In this way the DHA would be able to respond quickly and efficiently to changes in the resource base of its plans.

The availability of resources is not, of course, the only unpredictable factor facing DHAs. Other examples of uncertainty include policy changes by governments and breakthroughs in medical technology.

7.4   The Content of DHA Plans

In chapter 4 we mentioned that health authorities have to prepare two plans, namely strategic plans and annual programmes. In this section we outline in more detail the scope of these in DHAs. Strategic plans and annual programmes differ considerably in the amount of detail and precision. Consequently, some aspects are worthy of elaboration.

a. Strategic Plans

DHA strategic plans should begin with a review of the services in the district. Two important features would usually be included, first, the need for the various health services, and second, the existing level of service provided. Any disparity between the two sets of data would indicate that some change may be required. Health services in this context would usually be classified by the client group served. For example, the services for the elderly would include all the services provided for the elderly regardless of the way in which they are provided. In this way, all the services for a particular client group, whether provided by hospital or community services, can be considered comprehensively. A further more detailed analysis is by patient group. This is a sub-division of a client group. For example, the acute and general services are aimed at the broad client group requiring those services. This can be further analysed by such patient groups as those requiring orthopaedic services, or general surgery.

The development of a strategy for these client groups tends to cut across the unit management structure of a DHA. This unit structure is often subdivided into discrete departments which provide specific services. An example is the pathology department which will provide a service to most types of client group. To overcome this problem many DHAs established planning teams which as we mentioned earlier are orientated towards particular client groups and when combined represent a corporate approach to planning.

An important aspect of strategic plans is the assessment of the resources currently available to the DHA and a commentary on future resource forecasts. Thus the service shortfalls can be seen against the resources likely to be available to deal with them. Most DHAs will probably find themselves in the position of not having sufficient resources to overcome all of the identified problems and clearly priorities will have to be agreed. This process is the crux of strategic planning.

Reaching agreement on priorities can be a sensitive and painstaking matter. In essence, the task can be seen as selecting one client group as having a greater priority for resources than another. In practice, the choice is more complicated in that perhaps part of a client group may be given a high priority while the next priority may be part of another, unrelated client group. Hence the need for the more detailed analysis of patient groups. Some client groups may be so obviously deprived of resources that they can be ranked highly. Others may equally obviously be receiving an adequate share and can be ranked lowly. In between would almost certainly be the majority of client groups. This grey area is difficult to classify without local discussion and careful consideration. Because it is important to set out the basis of, and reasons for, selected priorities, such deliberations are essential ingredients of strategic plans. After the necessary consultation, a DHA should state which priorities it intends to rank highly over the next ten years, those which it does not intend to rank highly, and thirdly, those on which it may not have reached any decision at the time of preparing the plan, and which may be considered at a later date. A mere list of priorities and objectives in three categories would not suffice. If the plan is to serve any useful purpose in stimulating informed debate and explaining the choice of priorities, it must describe the reasons why each has found itself in its particular category.

Having identified, ranked and classified at least some priorities, the DHA will then have to state how it is going to tackle the problems. DHAs do not provide homogenous services, and specific proposals for change would almost certainly have to be expressed in terms of services related to client or patient groups. Analysing services in this way lends itself to the considera-tion of development options. For example, a proposal may have been agreed that more acute beds are required. Alternative schemes to imple-ment this proposal may include a new acute ward; a new geriatric ward to free existing acute beds or a contractual arrangement with private hospitals. Each may be effective in dealing with the problem, but may have vastly different implications. Again the DHA is faced with choice and it seems important once again to state in the strategic plan the reasons why pref-erences are expressed in a particular way. This should help in enabling others, such as the medical profession, the Community Health Council and the general public, to appreciate the basis of the DHAs proposed develop-ments.

A final element of the DHA's strategic plan could be its strategic pro-grammes. One programme of expenditure would be prepared for each allocation such as capital; revenue; joint financing, based on the forecast allocations. This would have important implications for the timing of solutions. Having identified the various resources likely to be available, these can be allotted to client groups. One way in which the process could work may be to take the highest priority, say a new DGH, and fix that in the programme. Various factors need to be considered and balanced, such as the earliest possible start date in contractual terms; the date by which it needs to be open; the availability of capital and revenue monies. These complicated, often conflicting, factors emphasise the need for strategic programmes in two respects: the need to weight the various constraints, and the need to look well ahead.

Having fixed the highest priority in the appropriate place and so on the resulting initial programme may not match the DHA's intentions exactly, and some fine tuning to the timings may be required before the programme can satisfy the DHA. Finally some form of contingency planning, perhaps using financial modelling, may be helpful in this respect.

Two interesting concepts are implied by this approach which is not recognised in many parts of the NHS. First is that the highest priority is not necessarily the first to be resolved. Planning lead times may mean that the highest priority may have to wait for a number of years before a solution can be implemented. This is particularly so when major capital schemes are involved. Such a priority, its solution and its timing, would not be lost sight of, but proposals of a lower priority may find their way into an earlier year of the strategic programme because of shorter lead time. Because they will be started earlier does not mean that they assume a greater priority. If there was a reduction in resources available, the main priority would not be deferred. Its position in the programme would remain fixed and the lower priority schemes would be adjusted around it. Secondly, the distribution of resources between client groups is not the result of some pre-determined distribution as envisaged by the national or regional guidelines. It arises from the implementation of the DHAs preferred selection of developments which in themselves are chosen by the DHA to overcome specific and identified problems of service provision. Thus the allocation of resources between client groups is a result of the strategy and not a pre-determined constraint on the DHA strategy.

DHAs begin the process of plan preparation by referring to the regional planning guidelines. When the completed strategies are seen by the RHA in a regional context, it could well accept the regional strategy as the sum of the DHA strategies. However, it would have to include an additional feature. The RHA's plan should include a commentary on the DHA's strategic plans particularly showing which national policies do not seem appropriate or are not being implemented.

A further aspect is a statement of those matters where the RHA and DHA required further discussions before agreement can be reached. National and regional discrepancies would probably fall under this heading, thus, by exception, indicating which aspects had been agreed.

b. Annual Programmes

Because annual programmes are derived directly from the appropriate strategic plan, it is tempting to assume that the content would be similar. The usual approach to annual programming seems to be that the appropriate years of the strategic plan are reviewed and restated in greater detail after reviewing matters such as resource forecasts, start and completion dates of capital schemes and service developments. One disadvantage with this view of an annual programme is that it disregards the nature of the plan. It is not meant to be merely a short term strategic plan. It is the means by which the strategic plan can be prepared for implementation through budgets of the DHA. The interposition of the annual programme between the strategic plan and the budgets exerts an influence on content of the budget. This seems to be the reasoning behind the annual programme preferred by the DHSS being in two parts. The first is the operational programme for the coming financial year, the second is the forward programme for the year after.

What should be the content of each of these programmes? Firstly, the operational programme should contain a minor capital programme and a draft revenue budget. The minor capital programme would include a list of those smaller capital schemes which need to be started or completed during the next financial year while the draft revenue budget would show which developments have to be financed next year, and which reductions and changes in service will be implemented. Two main types of development are, first, those that are service developments and would probably be mainly the recruitment of additional staff to expand current services. The second are the revenue effects of any new capital schemes that are due to be completed and commissioned in the next year. The RCCS methodology is helpful in this respect so that the items of additional cost can be readily identified. An example of a reduction in service would be the closure of a hospital, while, an example of changes in service would include a closure linked to rationalisation on another site.

Forward programmes do not require as much detail and firmness as operational programmes. All that is required is a list of planned proposals, in priority order, for that year. The proposals should of course bear relation to the forecast availability of resources and be consistent with the priorities expressed in the DHA's strategy. Because of the planning lead times it may be useful to extend the period of the forward programme from the single, second year of the operational plan to perhaps cover three, four or five years ahead. This should be accompanied by a commentary on the development of services envisaged.

A major feature of annual programmes is their proximity to reality. They should, therefore, be based on realistic and recent resource forecasts. The innate difficulties in preparing precise and accurate forecasts, even one year ahead, again justifies the use of contingency planning at this stage of the NHS Planning System. While its value in strategic planning may be challenged, it seems vital for annual programming if DMTs and DHAs are to respond quickly and sensibly to unexpected changes. The contents of annual programmes would therefore include an exploration of the alternative dates of implementation within the priorities set out in the strategic plan.

c. Joint Planning and Joint Finance

An important, but often neglected, item of both strategic and annual programmes is joint planning, and the related topic of joint finance. This needs particular mention. Perhaps the starting point is to draw the distinction between the terms. Joint planning is a statutory requirement for collaboration between DHAs and the respective local authorities, both county and district councils, in the use of the total resources available to the client groups in which each type of authority has an interest. Generally, they include the elderly, mentally handicapped, mentally ill and school children. The main thrust is an attempt to ensure that complementary services are planned and provided in such a comprehensive way that no potential clients are overlooked.

Joint financing is a catalyst for joint planning. As a separate allocation to DHAs, it represents NHS resources, mainly for social services but also for the eduction of disabled people and housing, which, under certain conditions, can be made available to both the DHA and the local authority to finance various projects, especially those which support the care in the community iniative. Having agreed a use for joint finance which offers DHA's benefits that will support their own plans, the proposals can then be expressed in the strategic and annual programmes.

7.5   Planning and the Financial Aspects

We would be the first to accept that finance is not the only aspect of planning nor is it necessarily the most important. Finance is only one of the resources available to DHAs and consequently planning must also concern itself with these other resources. The Bains Committee suggested that the resources available to local authorities could be classified into three types:

(a) Finance;
(b) Manpower;
(c) Land (including buildings).

We believe this analysis of resources applies equally to DHAs and this suggests a format for total planning, namely financial, manpower and land and buildings. Each of these three aspects is important to DHAs and we are probably all aware of examples of the consequences of failures to co-ordinate all three. For example, we have the new DGH which suffers a shortage of nursing staff due to inadequate preparation for nurse training or the health centre which cannot be built because the legal procedures surrounding land acquisitions had not been cleared early enough.

It is clearly beyond the scope of this book to deal with all aspects of health service planning and therefore the rest of this chapter will concentrate on the financial and economic techniques that can be used in planning. Although each of the three kinds of resource is important, we would emphasise the primacy of finance, for while we accept that the availability of finance does not automatically imply that other resources can be purchased, the absence of finance means that their acquisition is clearly not possible.

7.6 Techniques of Financial Planning

We would emphasise that none of the techniques to be outlined here are, in any sense of the word, new. They have been used with various measures of success by the private sector, and some parts of the public sector, for many years. What we have done is to examine each of these techniques and after briefly describing the principles underlying them we have discussed how they may be used for DHA planning purposes, and what amendments to the usual approach are needed if they are to be employed.

Simultaneously, we have given due consideration to the likely draw-backs and problems of using such techniques and have indicated some alternative approaches that may be adopted by DHAs. We must further emphasise that much of what we have written is not hypothetical. Some of these techniques have been used for a considerable period of time by a number of health authorities with whom we are familiar and their overall usage may be far greater than often envisaged.

We have already discussed how planning can vary in timescale. The relevance of each of these techniques depends upon the length of the planning timescale under consideration. Some of the techniques are far more relevant to strategic planning than to annual programming and this emphasis will be drawn out as appropriate. We now consider:

(a) Resource Forecasting;
(b) Programme Budgeting and Client Group Analysis;

(c) Investment Appraisal;
(d) Costing Systems;
(e) Financial Modelling.

7.7   Resource Forecasting

Strategic plans and annual programmes have to be prepared by DHAs on the basis of the resource and planning guidelines provided by the RHA. Included in these guidelines would be the RHA's view of the financial resources likely to be made available to the region and its view of how those resources would probably be distributed to DHAs over the period under review. In order to compile such a projection, the RHA will depend heavily on the Regional Treasurer. He will have at his disposal a range of information, the main sources being: DHSS advice; the present Government's policy: economic indicators; the RHA's approach to resource allocation. These factors are usually termed resource assumptions.

One of the most significant aspects of these guidelines, for the District Treasurer, is the information relating to the assumptions on which resource forecasts have been prepared. Forecasts of revenue and capital are usually made at constant prices, and so exclude the effects of any future inflation. Thus, they readily identify any projected growth or contraction of finance. This resource base of each DHA's strategic plan has important consequences for the pace of implementation of a strategy, and a careful assessment of the degree of optimism or pessimism reflected in the forecasts is essential. Such an assessment should be performed by District Treasurers in order to advise their fellow chief officers and the DHA of the scope for development or the need for retrenchment.

Some attempt must be made to deal with the range of uncertainty about these resource assumptions. Consequently the Treasurer may wish to vary the resource assumptions to reflect this uncertainty. Since the level of uncertainty increases in relation to the length of the planning timescale, the more distant resource assumptions will have a broader range than the nearer ones. Thus a wedge of resource forecasts, based on different forecasts, will result, with perhaps one forecast for the coming year with an increasing range for each of the subsequent years. This can be reflected in the DHA's strategy by producing alternative plans in line with the range of resource forecasts, while one could be selected as the most likely outcome, the remainder being contingency plans.

An alternative may be required where the District Treasurer does not consider the RHA's resource assumptions to be realistic or where there are no resource assumptions included in the planning guidelines. In this situation, the District Treasurer will need to make his own resource assumptions in order that he can make an assessment of the resources likely to be available to the DHA. The information available to him to do this will be the same as that available to the Regional Treasurer, mentioned previously.

Assumptions about Government policy are necessary in order to judge the extent to which the NHS as a whole will gain or lose in the PESC negotiations. For example, the Government's claims that the NHS is safe with them, and as being financially stable in relation to the level of public spending required by its economic policy. However, the sudden cash limit cuts announced by the Chancellor of the Exchequer in July 1983 followed by the manpower cuts seem to contradict such statements and conclusions have to be drawn about the Government's real intentions. Similarly, a view is required of the Government's use of the cash limits system and the adequacy of the inflation adjustment. For example, the prices addition for 1983/84 represented an average rise of some 5 per cent, proved to be realistic. However the similar sum for 1984/85 compares with predicted inflation at 7 per cent. The difference represents a real reduction in predicted resources, and the extent to which such effects are reflected in resource forecasts may be critical, especially for those DHAs scheduled to receive only limited growth.

The amount of growth planned for the NHS as a whole will greatly determine the pace of geographic equality. Similarly, the size of each RHA's development addition will determine the speed at which the DHAs will reach their target allocations. Projections as to the precise effect of these imponderables on the future revenue allocations are understandably tenuous and the Treasurer has the important role of assessing the adequacy and realism of the resource assumptions for his RHA or DHA.

The methods used by the RHA to finance developments can often be modified as demands and events change. For example, the method of holding specific reserves to finance the cost of the revenue consequences of medical appointments may change from one year to another. It may be necessary for a DHA to be able to respond to such changes as they arise, and the Treasurer has an important role in assessing the appropriateness of the RHA's financial methods, and the duration for which they can be maintained without modification.

Having examined and accepted or modified the resource assumptions for revenue and capital, the District Treasurer can turn his attention to the manpower assumptions included in the RHAs guidelines. The Treasurer will wish to assess their realism. This is especially important because most manpower forecasts in the NHS are not soundly based due to the extreme difficulty of aggregating unsound local data at national or regional levels. Consequently, the guidelines may not correspond with the DHA's view of the future manpower supply. For example, even if the national guidelines assume an increase in the number of nursing staff, the DHA might be aware of reasons why local recruitment of nursing staff might prove very difficult to achieve, for example by competition from private hospitals. However, one aspect remains dominant, namely, that the projected size of the DHA's labour force should be related to the revenue forecasts.

If the manpower cannot be financed from development additions, then a more difficult task must be undertaken. The DHA must decide if the finance can be provided from alternative sources, such as savings from other services. If no other sources can be found, then the DHA must consider if a limited recruitment for specific policy aims represents good value for money.

Many of the factors to be considered in preparing resource forecasts for a DHA can often be compensating. For example, it may be predicted that the Government will reduce the resources available for the NHS as a whole while the RHA may increase them significantly for the DHA. Conversely, the forecasts may combine to exacerbate the effect. Because the factors are varied and interact differently, great care has to be taken in constructing resource forecasts. We believe that it is extremely important to state clearly the assumptions on which such forecasts are based so that anyone using the data can be in no doubt as to its nature. In this way, the DHAs can formulate their plans in the knowledge that the resource base is necessarily a forecast and as such has innate limitations.

7.8   Programme Budgeting and Client Group Analysis

Programme Budgeting (PB) is an approach to planning rather than a technique. It was initially developed in the USA and first came to light following its introduction in the US Department of Defence and later in other US Federal Departments. Also, several US local authorities adopted a system of PB for the planning of their expenditure. PB came somewhat into vogue in Britain during the 1970s, especially in some local authorities, but it appears that its popularity has declined since then, as a consequence of the inherent difficulties of operating it successfully. Although the difficulties should not be dismissed lightly, in our opinion it is a 'technique' of great importance to health service planning and should be considered accordingly.

As a starting point for our discussions about PB, we refer back to the beginning of this chapter where we discussed the merits of corporate planning as opposed to departmental planning. It was argued that corporate planning was an approach which emphasised planning not along rigid departmental lines but for the health authority as a whole, based on its pre-determined objectives. As we state in Chapter 8, in the NHS, budgeting now involves the preparation of budgets along unit and departmental lines but since it is concerned mainly with the control of expenditure over one year, it cannot be regarded as a satisfactory aid to a system of corporate planning. Apart from the criticism of it as being too departmentally orientated, other criticisms can be levelled at the NHS approach to budgeting. These are discussed further in Chapter 8 but for the present we list some of them below:

(a) The one year period of budgets is generally too short a time to effect changes in the pattern of services.
(b) Budgeting tends to be incremental in nature. Budgets for a particular year tend to be based on the budget for the previous year, with adjustments made for marginal changes in departmental workload.
(c) Budgeting concerns itself only with what is spent on a service, namely the inputs, rather than what is produced in terms of better health, that is the outputs.

In an attempt to overcome these difficulties and to provide a system of budgeting which assists the planning process, PB was developed. Its analysis of the organisation's activities is complementary to corporate planning. It emphasises the preparation of budgets along corporate lines but also concerns itself with measuring the effectiveness of the organisations plans, as measured by the progress made in achieving objectives. Thus, PB is an aid to corporate planning. Having outlined the nature of PB we turn now to the main elements of a PB system. These can be described as being to:-

(a) determine the problems and needs of the community
(b) select priorities and set objectives to meet those needs
(c) prepare a programme structure
(d) classify existing activities by programmes
(e) develop and analyse alternative ways of meeting objectives
(f) evaluate and choose between alternatives
(g) classify planned activities by programme
(h) implement and monitor plans,
(i) review the efectiveness of activities
(j) feedback information for fresh decision making.

a. Determine the Problems and the Needs of the Community

This would involve a DHA in a considerable amount of investigatory work to establish the need for health services of its population. For example, it is necessary to establish the needs of the elderly, children, and mentally handicapped. Clearly this is a difficult task, but some attempt must be made by a series of investigations.

b. Select Priorities and Set Objectives

Once an assessment of needs has been made it will probably be found that the total needs of the community are very large, if not infinite, and furthermore, needs will differ greatly between different elements of the community. Since there is an obvious limit on resource availability, it will not be possible to meet all the needs. Consequently, it will be necessary for the DHA to select priorities showing which needs it will try to satisfy. From this, specific objectives will flow, showing to what extent the DHA will try to satisfy those needs. An important point here is that objectives must be expressed in terms of a defined and specified output. Objectives must not be expressed in terms of expenditure or manpower, i.e. inputs, but in terms of what we actually hope to achieve in the way of improved health, such as reduced mortality. Furthermore, objectives will be set according to client groups which we now describe.

c. Programme Structure

With PB, what we consider is not the health services themselves but the group in the community for whom these services are provided. The approach to planning would therefore be based on a consideration of all the services provided for a particular group, such as the elderly. It is desirable therefore that we identify the various groups in the community served by the DHA; then group the services accordingly. This is termed a programme structure. Such a programme structure has already been developed by the DHSS who consider the services as being run for eight 'client groups':

(i)   primary care services
(ii)   services for the elderly and physically handicapped
(iii)   services for the mentally ill
(iv)   services for the mentally handicapped
(v)   services for children
(vi)   maternity services
(vii)   general and acute services
(viii) other services.

There are, however, a number of problems with this programme structure. First it is an imperfect analysis. For example, the primary care services client group includes services which are not directed at the same type of clients, and would be more appropriately allocated to other client groups. Similarly, the general and acute services client group includes paediatrics, which could be classified as services for children. Furthermore, the acute and general group comprises about half of all DHA's expenditure. It is claimed by some that this client group is too large to be relevant for PB and should be disaggregated into a number of appropriate sub-groups. It is usually thought to be rather difficult to produce an accurate supporting financial analysis for a more detailed client group structure.

d. Classify Existing Activities by Programmes

Before considering the future, we must first see where we stand at present in relation to client groups. The next stage in PB must therefore be to take our present services which are usually classified by department and re-classify them according to the relevant client group which they serve. However, this is much easier said than done. It is difficult in practice to re-classify activities by client group since, as we have described, NHS accounting systems are functionally based and it is difficult to attribute expenditure to client groups. If developed further, specialty or patient costing could obviously assist in the task of assigning expenditure to client groups but for the present, DHAs need a simpler approach. Two possible methods which could be adopted by District Treasurers are to produce:

(i)   detailed studies of the costs incurred in an attempt to distribute them between client groups according to usage. For example, it would be necessary to break down the expenditure of the radiography department over client groups according to usage.

(ii) working assumptions to simplify the problem. This would result in broad apportionments of costs based on assumptions which may not have been validated.

Not surprisingly the DHSS sees the latter method as being the most generally applicable and some authorities have had success in using such methods. The basic approach is to utilise existing data, such as hospital costing returns and bed-use statistics for specialist hospitals such as geriatric and those for the mentally ill, in order to derive a cost per bed-day in those specialist hospitals. If we consider a DGH which treats patients from many client groups then we assume that the cost per bed-day already established for these client groups in the specialist hospitals is the same in the DGH. The remaining costs can be attributed to the acute and general services, Figure 8 is an example:

Figure 8– Example of a Calculation of Client Group Costs

Specialist Hospitals

Unit cost per bed-day — maternity	£40
Unit cost per bed-day — children	£35

A. DGH

Client Group	Bed-days	Unit Cost (£) from specialist hospital	Total Cost (£)
Total annual revenue expenditure			1,800,000
Less:			
Maternity	7,000	40	280,000
Children	10,000	35	350,000
∴ Acute and General Client Group expenditure			1,170,000

These are many objections to this procedure. For example, *are the DGH unit costs the same as specialist hospitals?* While this is unlikely, the differences are not considered to be significant for this purpose, although this has not been universally confirmed.

e. Develop and Analyse Alternative Ways of Meeting Objectives

This, of course, is the creative aspect of planning and all that can be said is that it is not sufficient to develop a single proposal as many feasible alternatives as possible must be generated. For example, improvements in peri-natal mortality might be brought about in a number of ways, perhaps by improved community care or by employing additional clinicians.

f. Evaluate and Choose Between Alternatives

Once we have generated alternatives, the next stage must be to evaluate them in terms of costs and benefits. In doing this we may utilise techniques such as discounted cash flow, cost benefit analysis and specialty costing. A choice between the alternatives must then be made, which will enable the DHA to meet its objectives.

g. Classify Planned Activities by Programme

Once we have considered the various alternatives and have decided which ones to implement, the next stage is to classify those planned future activities according to the client group analysis. The results will then be expressed as a corporate financial plan showing on which client groups the DHA intends to commit its resources in the future. The planning period here may vary but will be greater than one year ahead, and possibly up to ten.

h. Implement and Monitor Plans

If DHA plans are to be successful it is essential that they are implemented in the proper way and that expenditure is committed according to plan. Here then is the link with budgetary control. When the plan is to be implemented, the corporate financial plan can be turned into a conventional budget for implementation in the particular financial year.

i. Review the Effectiveness of Activities

This is perhaps the key aspect of PB: the measurement of how effective the DHA's activities have been in meeting its objectives. Since objectives would have been expressed in terms of output it is clearly necessary that actual achievement be measured in output terms.

For example, if one objective of a DHA was to reduce peri-natal mortality by a certain amount, then the measure of success of its activities, in achieving this objective, would be the actual reduction in mortality that took place. Output measurement is a complex subject and more will be said about it later in this chapter.

j. Feed back Information for Fresh Decision-Making

Actual achievement should be fed back to managers to enable fresh decisions to be made. This would provide information about those objectives achieved, and those not achieved.

If particular objectives were not achieved it would be necessary to reconsider the plans of the DHA in the hope of improving actual achievement in the future. Alternatively, the DHA might wish to consider whether the objective is truly feasible.

It will be observed that PB is much more than a budgeting technique in the usual sense. Traditionally, budgeting is concerned largely with the control of expenditure but PB is concerned with the planning of future activities. Perhaps the term programme *budgeting* is really a misnomer and a better term would be programme planning.

If PB is really such a useful tool of planning, it might be asked why it has not been more widely used by DHAs especially as it appears ideally suited. The answer is wrapped up in the difficulties of actually operating a system of PB and the two main difficulties can be described under the headings of (i) output measurement and (ii) complexity.

(i) Output Measurement The concept of the output of public services is important both for PB and other related activities such as cost benefit analysis. Many commentators have suggested that without output measurement, PB will lose much of its impact. In a commercial enterprise, measures of output are easy to devise, for example, tonnes of coal mined or number of cars produced, but the output of a DHA is far more difficult to define. The output of DHAs must be measured in terms of improved health or reduced sickness levels, the one being the converse of the other. However, this merely begs the question of how we measure the amount of health or sickness as there are no obvious measures. *When is a person sick or not not sick? Is A sicker than B and if so by how much?* Many attempts have been made to devise output measures for health services but little headway has been made.

(ii) Complexity It appears that wherever PB has been tried it has eventually been discarded in its pure form. This seems a harsh but unfortunately true judgement. The problem is that a system of PB comprises a series of complex and cumbersome procedures. For example, we have such matters as the assessment of needs; the classification into programmes; output measurement. It is easy to describe these in a few words but in practice each is extremely difficult to perform, and when aggregated into a system of PB, the difficulties are compounded.

While the DHSS has introduced a system of client groups for planning purposes which appears to be a PB approach, it is important to realise that the analysis is merely a broad apportionment of spending. It does not have the features of true PB. As DHAs are expected to comply with the financial analysis it is also important to distinguish the provision of data in a PB format with the operation of a system of PB. Because of the innate difficulties of PB, it seems almost impossible for it to be operated fully and successfully in a DHA.

7.9   Investment Appraisal

Like most organisations both in the private sector and public sector, health authorities have to make decisions about the amount of investment they should undertake and where that investment should be directed. Any assistance that can be given by the use of systems and techniques of investment appraisal will clearly be of benefit.

Investment appraisal is usually thought of as being applicable only to decisions about projects involving capital expenditure. Many capital projects are very expensive to undertake and decisions about them cannot easily be reversed. Furthermore, much of the additional revenue expenditure of the NHS is generated by capital schemes. For example, a new DGH usually leads to a large annual revenue commitment as a result of the need to employ additional staff or to purchase additional goods and services. Consequently, decisions about capital expenditure ultimately influence, to a great degree, the revenue expenditure of a DHA and therefore such decisions should be taken carefully. However, we would not wish to limit the use of investment appraisal to capital projects alone. We believe there are other situations where investment appraisal can be usefully applied:

a. Non-Recurring Expenditure

Much of the non-recurring funds of health authorities are spent on projects which although not strictly capital projects according to the NHS definition still involve expenditure of many thousands of pounds. Such projects can still be regarded as investment and hence should be subject to some form of investment appraisal.

b. Recurring Expenditure

We do not wish to get involved in semantic arguments but we believe that certain forms of recurring expenditure can be regarded as much an investment as capital expenditure. For example decisions about additional consultants are fairly irreversible and are likely to involve considerable additional recurring expenditure. Thus we believe some sort of systematic appraisal procedure should be applied to projects involving recurring expenditure.

c. Dis-investment

This can be regarded as the reverse of investment. In the present financial climate, many DHAs find it necessary to reduce their commitment in certain areas by, for example, closing hospital wards and/or whole hospitals. Again investment appraisal procedures can be applied to assist in deciding the best, or least damaging form of dis-investment.

The subject of investment appraisal has become topical in the NHS. In this section we wish to consider in some detail the topic of investment appraisal or as it is sometimes referred to, option appraisal. Initially we will consider two main approaches to investment appraisal namely those which employ the use of DCF techniques and those which employ the techniques of cost-benefit analysis (CBA). As well as describing the techniques and outlining their applicability to the NHS we will, of course, also point out their drawbacks. Although DCF and CBA may be of use to health authorities they can be regarded as nothing more than techniques which may form part of a much broader system of investment appraisal. Consequently at the end of this section we will consider investment appraisal in practice and will outline how a system of investment appraisal may be implemented and operated in a DHA.

a. Discounted Cash Flow

Traditional investment appraisal techniques such as the 'accountants rate of return' were used in the private sector of industry to ascertain whether it was financially opportune to invest in particular capital projects such as the construction of a factory. This was done by comparing the investment cost with the estimated additional cash flows that would be generated by the investment, to establish if the investment was worthwhile. The drawbacks of such techniques were that they ignored what is termed the 'time value' of money. They assumed that £100 received or paid in Year 2 was equivalent to £100 received or paid in Year 1, and that these amounts could be aggregated easily. Economics teaches in fact that this is not so. Money has a time value, and £100 received today is of greater value than £100 received in a year's time, since the £100 received now can be invested to produce an amount greater than £100 by the accrual of interest. Recognition of this fact led to the intoduction of DCF techniques for investment appraisal purposes.

It is not possible here to give a detailed description of the rationale of DCF techniques and the reader is referred to the many excellent texts on the subject. We do however, give a brief summary of the method. It is important that we take into account not only the size of the cash flows involved in projects but also the timing of them. Therefore, all the cash flows have to be expressed at a common point of reference. The usual way of doing this is by bringing all the cash flows to the present day by discounting them to give a present value of those cash flows. This assumes that the initial investment cost is at present value, while cash spent or received in a year's time has a different value because of the interest factor. So, £100 spent next year would have a present value of £90.91, assuming an interest rate of 10%. When conducting an appraisal of projects, the practice is to convert all cash flows to their corresponding present values. The financial viability of projects can, therefore, be assessed by a consideration of the net present value (NPV) of each of the projects. The NPV is merely the sum of the present values of the individual cash flows.

In the private sector, DCF techniques could be used to compare the revenues generated by an investment with the cost of that investment, all the cash flows being measured at the same point in time, namely the NPV. A positive NPV would imply that a project was profitable and hence worth going ahead with. A negative NPV would suggest that a project was not profitable and should not be implemented. In the public sector, and especially the NHS, capital investment is not usually of the kind that generates additional revenues. Investment is usually undertaken for social reasons such as improved health services. Conventionally, DCF techniques are concerned with indicating whether or not a project is likely to be profitable. Consequently, it is clear that discounting techniques cannot be used to decide whether major investments in the NHS should or should not be undertaken since profitability is not a valid measure of the value of a particular project. This does not mean, however, that DCF techniques are valueless in health authorities. We believe there are circumstances where they may be of use in defining the financial aspects of proposals. Consider, for example, the possible replacement of a hospital central heating system. It is clear that the primary decision here is whether or not to replace the system at the present time and we accept that such a decision will have to be based on managerial judgement. If management decides to replace the heating system, then this is not the end of the story since this now raises the secondary decision of what method of central heating should be employed *oil, coal, gas or electricity?* Each of these possible options will have different cost implications expressed in terms of initial investment, fuel costs, labour costs and maintenance costs, and clearly management will wish to know the overall cost of each option. Here then is a possible use for DCF techniques. If the annual running costs over the life of the system are discounted to present value and added to the initial investment the options could be ranked by order of overall NPV. The cheapest system will be the one with the lowest NPV. This is only one example but in any situation where there are several similar ways of implementing a policy then DCF techniques can be of use.

The present value of a cash flow, and hence the overall NPV of a project, clearly depends on the interest rate used. In DCF, the interest rate actually used is termed the discount rate. In the private sector, the choice of discount rate will be determined by the cost of capital, usually the interest rate at which finance can be obtained for capital investment. For health authorities, however, the choice of a discount rate is not clear cut. The most frequently recommended approach is to use the test discount rate (TDR) as formulated by HM Treasury. The rationale behind the TDR is that it represents the real rate of return sought by private companies on their marginal investments. Thus, it represents the rate of return foregone if resources were diverted from the private to the public sector. Currently the TDR is set at 5%. Unfortunately there are many arguments against health authorities using the TDR as a discount rate and indeed alternative rates have been suggested as being more satisfactory. Our conclusion, however, is that it is not possible to be definitive about the choice of a discount rate for the NHS. Arguments can be made for and against each of the suggested rates and it would be misleading to suggest that one particular rate is the correct rate. Often, the resulting NPV can vary depending on the rate used. Consequently, we suggest that health authorities should use a range of discount rates to test how sensitive to changes in discount rate is the ranking of project options. Obviously the rates advised by the DHSS and HM Treasury could be used in this range. It might be that all the discount rates used will give the same ranking of projects but alternatively, changes in the rate used might alter the ranking and thus a decision would need to be made about the choice of discount rate, and any differences in outcome interpreted.

b.   Cost Benefit Analysis (CBA)

We have described how DCF techniques have only limited use for capital investment appraisal in health authorities. The main reason for this was that DCF techniques are only concerned with cash flows whereas health authority investment decisions generally produce benefits other than the generation of additional revenue, namely the benefit of improved health services. However, other criticisms can be levelled at the use of DCF techniques for investment appraisal:

(i)   DCF techniques use a narrow definition of cost. They consider only accounting costs and ignore social costs.
(ii) DCF techniques do not take a long term view. They only consider projects during the period when cash flows are taking place, and do not consider the project over its complete lifespan.

One technique for overcoming these problems is CBA. It is a technique which has been used in the public sector to assist with decisions about major capital projects, but unfortunately it is fraught with difficulties and has many critics . The basic methodology of CBA can be summarised below:

(i)   Generate alternatives to the present situation.
(ii) List the costs and benefits of each alternative and of maintaining the existing situation.
(iii) Quantify those costs and benefits in physical terms.
(iv) Express the quantity of costs and benefits in monetary terms.
(v)   Discount costs and benefits to give a NPV for each alternative expressed as a net cost or net benefit.

This NPV can then be used as a basis for making a decision. Strictly speaking every project which shows a net benefit should be undertaken, but in practice, perhaps because of financial constraints this may not be possible and so a decision about which projects to undertake may still be required. In strict CBA terms, the project with the greatest net benefit would be preferred.

Unfortunately, the problems of CBA seem almost insurmountable. While it may be possible to list the various costs and benefits, it may prove very difficult to reach agreement as to how to quantify them and it becomes even more difficult to put a monetary value on the physical quantities of cost and benefits. The CBA methodology frequently requires a monetary value on such factors as noise, comfort, time and even human life.

In spite of its limitations, we wish to consider the possible applications of CBA in health authorities – and in this context we can consider two possible approaches. One is specifically related to narrow economic objectives; the benefits to be derived from health care are assessed only by reference to the extent to which it results in an increased gross domestic product (GDP) due to the improved health of the working population. The methodology of such an approach has been discussed in other publications, but can be expressed in a simple form below:

(i)   Estimate, for future years, the likely increase in working time, due to a reduction in sickness, if a particular health service policy is adopted.
(ii) Express this in monetary terms using gross average earnings.
(iii) Discount the additional earnings to give a NPV.
(iv) Compare this with the costs of the policy to decide whether implementation is worthwhile.

There are of course many objections to such a narrow approach to the measurement of benefits. For example, it is clear that improved health might be only one determinant of improved productivity and it would then be necessary to try to separate out the effects of improved health from other factors. Also there is the problem as to the extent to which expenditure by health authorities actually improves health directly; other causes of improvement might be better housing or improved sanitation. However, the main objection to this approach concerns the morality of measuring benefits, and hence making decisions, only be reference to these narrow economic objectives. By these criteria no resources would ever be devoted to the aged, the infirm or the mentally handicapped as they contribute little to GDP. For similar reasons it would appear that little would be spent on improving the standard of health of housewives or the unemployed. These implications would be unacceptable to most people and therefore we conclude that the pure economic approach must be rejected as inappropriate.

The alternative approach to CBA is to attempt to take a much wider view of the benefits of health services. The implications of such an approach are that factors such as absence of pain and distress, general relief from sickness, longevity of life and improved health as well as the more material benefits such as the productive capacity of working individuals would be brought together. The difficult issue concerns the relative values to be attached to these benefits.

If we decide to adopt this broader approach to CBA, this raises the problem of how we measure the benefits of health services. *How do we measure the benefits of relieving pain or the benefit of preventing mental deficiency in children?* Even more, perhaps, *how do we measure the benefit of saving life, both the benefit to the person whose life is saved, and the benefit to the community?* This problem of measuring the 'output' of health services is an exceedingly difficult one, as we have already seen in the earlier section on PB.

If we are to adopt this approach to CBA then the following must be known:

(i) *How do we measure, in physical terms, the output and benefits of particular packages of health care?*
(ii) *How do we decide whether one volume of output is better than another, and if so by how much is it better?*

Clearly it is very difficult, if not impossible, to measure many of the benefits that will accrue from the sorts of investments carried out by health authorities. Furthermore, we believe it is less than honest to suggest that at some time in the future, with sufficient research being done, we will be able to quantify and value the output of such investments. We believe that a simpler approach to CBA should be adopted. The advantage of using CBA for investment appraisal purposes is that it forces the decision-maker to generate alternatives and to consider the costs and benefits of those alternatives. We believe this can still be done without the need for quantification and valuation. Consequently, we believe the following approach to CBA might be usefully employed by health authorities:

(i)	Identify the priorities and objectives of the authority;
(ii)	Identify any constraints on action such as financial or manpower;
(iii)	Generate alternatives to the present situation in the light of the informaiton in (i) and (ii);
(iv)	Forecast the financial costs (or savings) of each alternative both capital costs and running costs;
(v)	Discount these financial costs to give a NPV for each alternative;
(vi)	Identify the benefits of each alternative and quantify where possible (but not necessarily in monetary terms);
(vii)	Identify any non-financial social costs;
(viii)	Present the relevant information on each alternative to the decision-maker.
(ix)	The decision maker makes an explicit subjective decision about which alternative(s) to implement;
(x)	Some time after implementation, review the success or failure of the investment.

The advantage of this approach is that each alternative has been thoroughly examined to identify the costs and benefits, both financial and social. The financial costs of each alternative have been converted to a single NPV to simplify the information presented. On the basis of this information a subjective decision will be made. Although this approach to CBA does not have the pseudo-scientific precision of a full CBA study, it does have the following advantages:

(i) Alternative approaches are considered.
(ii) Costs and benefits of each alternative are identified and examined.
(iii) Information is presented in a simple form.
(iv) The procedures involved are relatively simple and hence cheap.

We must emphasise, however, that what is described above is nothing more than the bare bones of an approach to investment appraisal in a health authority. it is a much more complex task to actually implement a system of investment appraisal based on the above method. The task of implementation is discussed overleaf.

c. Limitations of Investment Appraisal Techniques in the NHS

Having discussed the possible applictions of DCF and CBA techniques in
the NHS, we now summerise some of their overall limitations and drawbacks. Broadly speaking these can be summarised under two main
headings; subjectivity and inappropriateness.

(i) Subjectivity It appears that one aim of these techniques is to introduce
some degree of objectivity into the decision-making process of health
authorities. It was to be hoped that the use of these techniques could in
some way reduce the degree of subjectivity inherent in most investment
decisions. Unfortunately, the very use of these techniques still involves a
great element of subjectivity. For example:

(i)   the choice of discount rate
(ii) the method of assessing benefits
(iii) the forecasting of costs.

Consequently we must ask whether these techniques really do improve
the decision-making process or whether they are just pseudo-objective,
giving an impression of scientific precision and rationality where it does
exist.

(ii) Inappropriateness We use the term inappropriateness to indicate that,
even if objectivity were achieved, the decisions arrived at by the use of these
techniques might not be the correct ones from the point of view of the
health authority although it might be correct from the point of view of the
country as a whole.

To see why this is so, we need first to recap a little on the method of
financing the NHS. It will be recalled from earlier chapters that health
authorities receive annual allocations of money; a revenue allocation and
a capital allocation. If we consider the capital allocation, we can see that to
the health authority, capital might be regarded as a 'free good'.

To understand this, let us first consider the position of say a local
authority or a water authority. These organisations usually have to borrow
funds to finance capital expenditure and these funds have ultimately to be
repaid with interest. This means they have to bear an annual debt charge
for the repayment of the loan. This, however, is not the case in a health
authority. Once capital expenditure is incurred, it is over and done with,
there is no ongoing annual charge for the use of capital. Furthermore, if the
health authority does not fully use its capital allocation, then apart from a
limited amount of carry-forward and virement to revenue, the unspent

portion is lost. The result of this approach to capital funding is, that health authorities have no incentive to minimise capital spending. If capital expenditure is incurred, there is no annual debt charge to be borne, and if it is not incurred, the unspent portion of the capital allocation will be lost.

For example, consider now the position of a health authority faced with the following investment options:

Table 8 – Example of Investment Options

	Option A		Option B	
	£	£	£	£
Capital Cost		300,000		500,000
Revenue Cost per annum	80,000		50,000	
for five years	80,000		50,000	
	80,000		50,000	
	80,000		50,000	
	80,000	400,000	50,000	250,000
Total cost		700,000		750,000
NPV of costs (including capital costs)		628,320		705,200

For simplicity, both options are identical in all other aspects other than cost. Consequently, a decision must be made on the basis of cost. The rational economic decision suggests that option A is the more appropriate as it shows the lowest present value of costs when discounted at a TDR of 5%. Acceptance of option A would ensure that the total costs to the public sector are minimised. Suppose, however, that the health authority is in a financial position where capital funds are plentiful but revenue finance is limited. From the point of view of the health authority, it might be better to adopt option B, as in this way it minimises its use of its scarce revenue funds.

Furthermore, as we have already said, since capital is a 'free' good there will not be an additional burden of debt charges. Thus it is the case that the unusual system of financing health authority's capital expenditure leads to a situation where the financial practice of health authorities can contradict the needs of the community as a whole.

d. Project Appraisal in Practice

While we believe that health authorities should use some form of appraisal technique on the lines set out in this section, it is not common practice to do so.

Health authorities have been expected to follow procedures which have as an important feature the explicit public choice between options for capital schemes. The public demonstration of the choice would involve members of health authorities who will be able to play an active part in taking decisions.

The appraisal of the options would include the following:

(i) Definition of objectives showing how the proposed development relates to the health authorities' stated strategy.

(ii) Consideration of the main options for meeting the service objectives.

(iii) Identification, evaluation and timing of the costs and quantifiable benefits of each option, which would include; the estimated capital costs, plus land; RCCS; significant quantifiable costs imposed on other public bodies, the private sector and individuals; quantifiable revenue savings and benefits.

(iv) Social benefits explicity set out for each option.

(v) Discounting as has been outlined previously in this chapter.

We see this approach as being a significant development for Treasurers. In our view, they should assume responsibility for co-ordinating the appraisal work in their authorities, and as such will take personal responsibility for aspects such as quantifying costs and benefits and discounting. No other chief officer will be better suited for the co-ordinating role.

What has been said above and earlier is little more than an outline as to how investment appraisal might be applied in a health authority. it is not always appreciated that more work is required to actually implement a working system of investment appraisal in a health authority. Recent work has shown that investment appraisal is a three stage process:

(i) Initial Appraisal Each year an in-depth initial appraisal of projects will be carried out to decide what should be included in the authority's annual programme. This initial appraisal will consider the various options available to the authority and the end product will be a list of planned development projects in order of priority.

(ii) Final Appraisal Once the authority has a firm indication of the resources available to it, the final appraisal will be carried out. Projects included in the operational plan will be reviewed in the light of up-to-date cost estimates and any major changes in circumstances which might affect the priority of development projects.

(iii) Past Implementation Review. At some suitable time after the chosen option has been implemented it is necessary to carry out a review of the

success of the project. This should establish how far the intended claimed objectives have been achieved and any collective action that may be necessary.

It is beyond the scope of this book to outline the detailed steps of the investment appraisal procedures, but the main features are listed below:

(i)   DMT circulate to UMGs detais of the DHAs priorities and objectives and any constraints on action such as financial constraints.

(ii)   UMG consults within unit and develops a list of proposed development projects and any alternatives.

(iii)   Treasurer costs out these proposed development projects and computes a NPV at a range of discount rates.

(iv)   UMG identifies the likely benefits of proposed projects.

(v)   UMG ranks proposed projects in priority order and submits this ranking and all relevant information to the DMT.

(vi)   DMT considers priority rankings from all units and prepares a district-wide priority listing of projects. This listing would then be incorporated in the DHA operational plan.

(vii)   Prior to the commencement of a financial year, a final appraisal is performed and the decision is made about which projects should be implemented in the year.

(viii) Sometime after projects have been implemented, a post-implementation review is performed. This would cover both the costs and benefits of the project.

What is shown above is only the bare-bones of the system. The detailed procedures are necessarily complex and require certain checks and balances as well as a considerable degree of decision making to be delegated to UMGs.

7.10   Costing Systems and Planning

In recent years it has been recognised that cost information has a much broader relevance in health authorities than merely for the production of hospital cost booklets. Cost information has relevance to decision making about resource allocation, monitoring and, especially relevant to this section, planning decisions. In this section we shall look at the different types of costs information that must be produced to see its relevance to planning. Costing is topical at present in view of the recommendations of Working Party F of the Korner Committee on what types of financial information health authorities should be producing.

To avoid confusion, one point is clarified immediately, namely our use of the term costing. It is often used in the NHS to describe the annual cost statements. However, this is not what we mean by costing. Our interpretation is the continuous analysis of the existing cost of DHA activities. Thus, our definition of costing is a dynamic one which is concerned with the use of cost accounting systems to provide cost information for decision making at any time, not just after the year end.

Within a particular unit of a DHA, for example, a hospital, the usual approach to costing is a departmental one. The essence of this approach is that details about the various financial transactions, for example, wage payments, and stores issues, are recorded against relevant hospital cost centres. Thus, costing information is available about the expenditure of these particular departments. Examples of typical departmental cost centres are:

(a) Nursing
(b) Physiotherapy
(c) Radiography
(d) Pharmacy
(e) Catering.

In this way, the costing system is able to provide information, at any time, about the expenditure of the hospital, on nursing, physiotherapy, etc. In practice, the system will probably be able to provide more specific information. Thus, for example, as well as showing the total nursing expenditure, the system might well provide an analysis of nursing expenditure by ward and theatre.

It will be noticed that with this form of costing, the focus of concern is the hospital department and not the patient. Costing systems are designed to produce information about the running costs of hospital departments and not about the overall costs of actually treating patients. The consequence of this approach to costing is that very little information is available about the cost structure of health services expressed in terms of clinical activities. Thus, for example, little or no information is available about the overall cost of treating different diseases or conducting various surgical operations.

An alternative to collecting information about hospital departments is to collect it about patients or groups of patients. This alternative approach might be termed patient-orientated cost information.

In its report, Working Party F of the Korner Committee suggested four possible ways in which such patient-orientated cost information might be produced:

(a) Specialty Costing
(b) Diagnostic Group Costing

(c) Clinical Team Costing

(d) Patient Costing

Each of these different approaches is discussed below.

a. Specialty Costing

This is perhaps the best known of the four approaches listed and is based on the original research of Professor Charles Magee of Cardiff University.

In a project based at the Bridgend General Hospital, procedures were developed which enabled the revenue expenditure of the hospital to be re-classified along specialty lines.

Whereas the day-to-day costing system of the hospital classified expenditure by department, such as nursing, pharmacy, pathology, this project provided a breakdown of total hospital expenditure between in-patient services and out-patient services. A further breakdown of in-patient expenditure provided an analysis between medical specialities. The results of this are summarised in Table 9:

Table 9 – Specialty Costs of Bridgend General Hospital

		£'000	£'000
Total expenditure for 1978/79 consisting of:			4,642.7
a)	Inpatients:		
	(i) General Medicine	557.6	
	(ii) General Surgery	636.8	
	(iii) Geriatric	362.7	
	(iv) Opthomology	105.4	
	(v) Paediatric	195.5	
	(vi) Obstetric/Gynaecology	614.5	
	(vii) Orthopaedic	403.7	
	(viii) Dermatology	9.8	
	(ix) Rheumatology	16.1	2,902.1
b)	Outpatients		583.9
c)	Casualties		182.6
d)	Services for general practitioners		83.6
e)	Undistributed costs		890.5

To enable such a re-classification of expenditure to take place, it is necessary that techniques are developed to enable the expenditure of hospital departments to be analysed over medical specialties. Thus, for example, the expenditure of the pathology department would be analysed over the medical specialties according to the use made, by each specialty, of that service. Doing this for all hospital departments enables an overall specialty cost to be built up.

Since the original work at Bridgend, the procedures developed have been replicated several times in a series of pilot studies thus proving the feasibility of performing specialty costing in DHAs. Furthermore there are a number of DHAs who have on their own initiative produced a specialty analysis of expenditure. Thus the approach is now well developed.

The major problem, however, with the above approach is the lack of flexibility. The present functional approach to NHS costing can be rightly criticised on the grounds that it is inflexible in that the costing system produces only one kind of information, namely functional. To set up a system that produces only specialty cost is merely to continue that inflexibility. Furthermore, we believe that medical specialities are not particularly homogenous in nature. The activities of a medical specialty can be quite diverse, ranging from the very simple to the complex. Consequently producing information on the costs of specialties tends to disguise a wide variation in the cost of providing medical care. For example, producing information of the cost per patient of an orthopaedics specialty would disguise the fact that some patients are treated for minor ailments and receive simple and cheap treatment, while other patients receive a complete course of treatment which is very expensive.

b. Diagnostic Group Costing

This approach, also referred to as disease costing, would overcome some of the problems of lack of homogeneity of specialties referred to above. Instead of regarding the medical specialty as the cost centre and capturing data about the costs of running medical specialties we go one stage further and regard a specific diagnostic group as the cost centre. Thus it is necessary by means of various allocations and apportionments, to discover the running costs of each diagnostic group. Then diagnostic group costing would identify the costs of specific clinical conditions, within that specialty, of cardiology, virology etc.

c. Clinical Team Costing

This approach is not so much directed at the patient as at the clinician actually treating them. The aim is not so much to establish the costs incurred by a patient or group of patients but rather the costs incurred by a group of clinicians within a specialty. Clinical team costing is usually thought of in conjunction with some form of specialty budgeting and this is discussed further in Chapter 8.

d. Patient Costing

The final approach to be considered is one where the cost centre is the individual patient and information is collected about the costs of treating and maintaining every patient.

The importance of this approach to costing is not that managers need information about the costs of individual patients but that if a file of patient costs is held on computer it would be a simple task for the data to be aggregated in different ways to produce a variety of information. A number of indicators could be attached to each patient such as: disease classification; specialty; consultant; method of treatment; and the computer could then group patients together to produce information such as:

(a) the costs of running a medical specialty
(b) the cost of treating a disease
(c) the costs incurred by a clinical or team of clinicians
(d) the differing costs of treating the same disease by different methods.

The number of types of information to be produced is limited only by the number of 'indicators' used. Thus, by going down to the level of the individual patient, maximum flexibility can be maintained and cost information produced on a variety of bases other than just the specialty base.

The total costs attributed to a patient comprise the various individual costs of accommodating, treating and feeding the patient. Consequently separate charges must be recorded against each patient to reflect the cost of performing various 'events' on their behalf. The term 'event' is used to describe a range of activities needed to maintain patients in hospital. Examples are:

(a) pathology – tests performed on patients;
(b) wards – nursing care performed for patients;
(c) pharmacy – drugs prescribed to patients.

To record total patient costs it is necessary to set pre-determined charges for each of the possible 'events'. These would include, for example, a charge per test and a charge per drug. As 'events' are performed for patients the appropriate charge will be recorded. In this way, data will be built up about the total costs of treating different patients. Information about particular patients or groups of patients can be extracted as desired.

It is worth noting that such systems of patient costing have only become feasible since the revolution in micro-computing which has radically reduced the cost of computing facilities.

e. The Systems Compared

In this section we have attempted a brief comparison of the merits of the four approaches discussed above. Basically the four approaches must be judged according to two main criteria:

(a) cost of setting up and maintaining the system
(b) usefulness to management.

Specialty costing is now a relatively well-developed approach to costing which has been tried in a number of health authorities. The costs of setting up the system and maintaining the system are said to be relatively modest[10.] Against this, however, there must be considerable doubts as to the use made of the information. After considerable study we are still not convinced that such specialty costing information will have much direct use to managers. We must emphasise that there is no benefit in just comparing specialty costs between hospitals if no action is then taken because of a lack of back-up information. Specialty costing may be used as an input to specialty budgeting and this is discussed further in Chapter 8.

Patient costing is undoubtedly less developed and less well-tried than specialty costing. The costs of setting up and maintaining such a system are undoubtedly greater than for specialty costing where the DHA started from scratch.

However, such costs must be judged alongside two developments in NHS computing which would undoubtedly simplify and hence cheapen the cost of patient costing systems:

(i) the growth of patient administration systems in DHAs
(ii) the existence of micro-computing facilities in DHAs.

Given the untried nature of patient costing it is clearly only possible to speculate as to the usefulness of such systems. We believe, however, that patient costing will ultimately prove to be the best approach to costing because of the inherent flexibility. As previously mentioned, a patient costing system could produce specialty costs, disease costs, clinical team costs plus a whole range of additional information. Thus a patient costing system is able to cope with changing managerial needs over a period of years.

The other two approaches to costing we regard as something of half-way house approaches in that they would prove more complex to introduce than specialty costing without achieving the full flexibility of a patient costing system. Thus they must be judged with caution.

Finally this section would be incomplete without a mention of the recommendations of the Korner Working Party F. Their report concluded that although patient costing would ideally be the best approach it could not be regarded as practical for early implementation *across* the NHS. On the other hand the report concluded that specialty costing could provide, at moderate cost, a considerable improvement in the financial information produced and should therefore be introduced across the NHS.

f. Variable and Fixed Costs

Another major weakness of current NHS costing systems is their difficulty in distinguishing between variable costs and fixed costs. By fixed costs we mean those which are totally fixed in relation to the activity of the organisation and by variable costs we mean those which vary with the level of activity.

Using a hospital as our example, if extra patients are admitted to hospital then it will be necessary to feed them, prescribe drugs, etc., and so additional expenditure will actually be incurred which would not have been incurred if they had not been admitted. These types of costs (food, drugs, etc.) are termed variable costs. Consider now the rates bill or the heating costs of the hospital. These will remain the same whether the additional patients are admitted or not and these types of costs are termed fixed costs. In any organisation it is our belief that an appreciation of how different elements of cost respond to changes in activity, is one of the most important facts managers need to grasp. Therefore in setting up a costing system it is important that we give some indication of which costs are fixed costs and which are variable costs, in relation to the activity level of the hospital as measured by patient activity.

The snag of course, is that some costs may be both fixed and variable depending on particular circumstances. For example, if additional patients enter a ward it may be necessary to employ an additional nurse and hence nursing is, in this case, a variable cost. However, these additional patients can usually be accommodated within the existing nursing establishment and in this situation nursing is therefore a fixed cost.

Consequently, a desirable feature of a costing system is that it should distinguish between those costs which are definitely variable and those which are normally fixed. Figure 9 illustrates the distinction.

Figure 9 – Distinction between some Variable and Fixed Costs

Definitely Variable	*Normally Fixed*
Drugs	Nursing labour costs
Pathology consumables	Medical labour costs
Catering provisions	Pathology labour costs
Sterile packs	Radiography labour costs
	Catering labour costs

Our conclusion, therefore, is that the best type of costing system for DHAs is one that records patient costs and which distinguishes between fixed and definitely variable costs. It is not suggested, however, that such a costing system would replace the departmental system as this would still be required as a component of budgetary control. What it would do is supplement the departmental system by providing a broader range of information for decision making.

g. The Uses of Costing Information

We now turn to the uses that can be made of patient or specialty costing information. As will be seen from other chapters, the kind of information that could be produced would have value for resource allocation and financial control procedures but in this chapter we shall concentrate on its uses in planning. We believe there are three main uses:

(i) RCCS If a DHA decided to proceed with a major capital project, finance will be needed to meet the annual running costs of the hospital, such as medical and nursing salaries, drugs and provisions. These are usually termed the RCCS, and it is vital that DHAs have reliable estimates of the likely RCCS resulting from capital developments. The absence of such information could mean the DHA finding itself short of revenue finance and unable to open the hospital on time. The usual method of forecasting RCCS is by means of a formula called the 45 sample hospitals' formula. This approach is regarded by many as being unsatisfactory and locally produced cost information about the running costs of medical specialties or sub-specialties might be an improvement and will certainly be more appropriate.

(ii) Resource Re-allocation The alert DHA will be one which does not assume that a particular pattern of service provision will be satisfactory at all times. It will recognise that factors such as demographic and social changes are continually occurring and thus the pattern of health services must change with it. For example, it may recognise that increasing unemployment may lead to greater psychiatric illness and consequently more resources will need to be devoted to services for the mentally ill. In the past such changes in the pattern of services could usually be financed by the use of development monies but the constraints on public expenditure in recent years have restricted this practice. Consequently in the event of little or no additional finance being made available to the NHS, DHAs will have to

manage with what they have got. Service developments in one area will have to be financed by means of reductions in other areas or increased efficiency. In the event of such re-distribution being considered, the first thing DHAs will wish to know is how much finance will be released by contracting one clinical activity and how much will be absorbed by expanding another. Consequently it will be desirable for them to have access to financial information about clinical activities distinguishing between variable costs and fixed costs. Using this information, an assessment of the financial effects of any resource re-allocation can be made.

(iii) Opportunity Costs Perhaps the most important facet of health service planning is a recognition that resources are finite and that each course of action undertaken implies many other courses of action foregone. For example, each heart transplant performed implies the foregoing of, for example, a number of hernia operations and hip replacements. This consideration of opportunities foregone is known to economists as the opportunity cost concept. Currently, decisions about the commitment of health service resources are made, to a large degree, without any knowledge of the costs of the various options under consideration. We are not suggesting that such decision be made purely on the basis of cost but merely that cost information should be made available to the decision maker who will then make what is ultimately a subjective decision given the knowledge of cost. For example, the presentation of information to decision makers that each heart transplant costs say ten times as much as each pacemaker implant might be an unpalatable fact, but is essential for rational decision making. The problem, of course, is that the required information is not currently available but the development of patient costing system could rectify this deficiency.

(iv) Performance Indicators. Cost information can also be used as a measure of performance of individuals or departments. These are dealt with in Chapter 5.

7.11   Financial Modelling

A model is a simplified approximation of a particular situation in the real world. The model will be constructed from the essential and significant features of that real world. Models, financial or otherwise, are not replicas. Some features of the real world are so important that they must be included in the model. Conversely, some features may be so trivial as to be readily discarded without affecting the model's validity. By omitting these elements, the 'essential and significant' features of the real world remain.

A key principle of modelling is validation. If a financial model produces results which do not correspond closely enough to the situation it represents, then the model must be restructured or discarded. Many excellent publications dealing with financial modelling already exist, and readers are referred to these for further information.

As a technique, financial modelling has been practised in principle for many years by asking the question *"what if. . . ?"*. With the advent of the computer, particularly the cheaper micros, and software packages, sophisticated financial modelling has become feasible. This allows a greater number of alternative proposals to be considered and also improves the precision of the financial evaluation of those options. Against this background, we have described some of the situations in the NHS where financial modelling techniques can be applied.

Beginning with a relatively simple example, modelling can be used to forecast the levels of resources over the strategy period. If the District Treasurer was not too sure about the future resources available to the DHA, he could construct a simple model which could take the current year's revenue allocation and extend it over the strategy period by specified annual growth rates. To test various assumptions, a different growth rate could be used, either for the whole period or for selected years. By taking a similar view with other resources, such as capital and joint finance, the whole resource base of the DHA's strategy can be quickly and easily reviewed.

In isolation, such a task could be completed quickly by using a desk calculator. However, when it is linked with the planned spending of those resources, the model becomes too complex to handle without a computer.

For example, the DHA may wish to consider the implications of the resulting ten-year spending programmes arising from alternative strategies. Before advice can be prepared on these matters, the District Treasurer would need to prepare the two programmes within the constraint of the resource forecasts. If a model had been constructed which held details of all possible developments, and their associated revenue and capital costs for the strategy period, it would be relatively easy to select those developments which coformed to each alternative strategy and include those in draft spending programmes. By including the resource forecasts in the model, a comparison can be made and further modifications made to the draft programmes. After the DHA has selected its preferred strategy and programme, subsequent changes, in factors such as costs and resources can be easily monitored and assessed.

A more complicated application of modelling is in respect of a particular schemes or development to be included in such programmes. For example, the DHA may be considering the provision of a new DGH, and an assessment will be required of the RCCS, both the total amount and the phasing, Such calculations are usually complex and time consuming and when completed are not easy to amend. Modelling can be of assistance by enabling one to vary each of the factors involved in the calculation of RCCS to see what would be the overall effect.

The information requirements of models such as this are often very precise. In particular, the unit costs of each type of staff to be employed in the new DGH is required, together with unit costs of the various types of patients to be provided for. An assessment of matters such as staffing levels, patient throughput and workload are required for each department, ward and clinic of the DGH. Such spurious precision in the basis of estimates, may result in an inaccurate total picture when combined, and it is in this respect that modelling can help. When the RCCS are being considered, those estimates which are not sufficiently accurate can quickly be varied and a revised total calculated. Similarly, as costs increase due to wage awards and price increases, the effects can be reflected by using the model.

One final example of an application that we wish to include is in relation to the proposals for changes in related services with totally different costs. Consider the possibility of transferring the care of some of the elderly from hospital services to community services. Many people consider that such a proposal would prove to be cheaper and more desirable. By using a model, the various units costs can be combined with the likely levels of workload, and the proposal can be evaluated in financial terms. This type of model can be extended to produce a model of the activities of the DHA as a whole or in part.

Two common requirements can be discerned in the last two examples of more complex models. They are the need for unit costs and workloads. Without such information in a reliable form it is generally not possible to construct valid complex models. Examining unit costs first, these are built into models so that the financial effect of changes, either actual or planned, can be established. Assume, for example, that one simplified element of a model is that for each patient in a new DGH, five pathology tests are carried out. In order to quantify the pathology costs of the DGH, the cost of each test is required. By applying the unit cost of an average test, the required information can be generated. Once the relationship between a test and the unit cost has been established, the effect on overall expenditure of changes in the unit cost can be easily calculated by using modelling techniques. A financial model can comprise several such relationships, and be used in a relatively quick and easy way to calculate and assess the effect in total of a series of individually small changes.

The same effect can be seen with workload information. Using the same example, it is important to know first, how many patients of the various types there will be at any one time, and second how many and what type of tests will be required for the different patients. Having established a measure of the workload, and incorporated this into a model, it is a simple task to ask the computer for an assessment of the effect of changes in the overall workload, either in total or in part.

When these two variables of unit costs and workload are combined, the possible changes that can be modelled become numerous. Because such facilities are readily available, it is tempting to assume that the results are valid, and it is in this respect that modelling should be embarked upon with great caution. It is vital that postulated relationships between the variables of unit cost and workload are validated to ensure that they adequately reflect the actual situations. This may be obvious in some cases. For example, one doctor may prescribe drugs and he will incur a higher unit cost than another doctor who prescribes less expensive drugs or smaller quantities of the same drug. In such cases, one tendency to avoid is to assume that a general, average relationship exists everywhere at all times and hence can be expressed directly in a model. The assumption may be a serious distortion of the actual situation, and could result in the eventual output of the model being unrealistic and inaccurate. If such broad assumptions are prevalent in a model, the results could be so inaccurate as to be valueless.

8

Financial Control in
District Health Authorities

8.1 Aspects of Financial Control

The Treasurer of a health authority is responsible for the control of the authority's finances and should, therefore, supervise the instruments of internal financial control. However, financial control should go beyond the mere satisfying of the Treasurer's responsibility, and emphasis should also be placed on the effectiveness and efficiency of the authority's activities. The various aspects of financial control that we shall consider in this chapter can be grouped as follows:

(a) Budgeting and Budgetary Control
(b) Costing Information
(c) Internal Audit.

8.2 Structure of Budgetary Control in DHAs

Any textbook on budgetary control will ascribe the following main aims for budgetary control in organisations:

(a) Delegation – by giving managers a budget, the organisation is delegating authority to the budget holders to spend up to the limit of the budget.
(b) Planning – the budget is a form of organisational plan for one year expressed in financial terms.
(c) Control – budgetary control is a mechanism for ensuring that the organisation achieves the planned levels of service and expenditure.
(d) Motivation – budgetary control systems can motivate budget holders to achieve better managerial performance.

Like all large organisations, health authorities have systems of budgetary control designed to achieve the above aims. Since 1982 the form of budgetary control operating in most health authorities is referred to as unit budgeting. The precise arrangements will obviously vary between DHAs but we discuss here the usual practice.

It was mentioned in Chapter 1 that responsibility for the day-to-day management of a unit such as a hospital, or a group of hospitals, falls upon the UMG. This management structure will clearly have implications for the operation of budgetary control in DHAs. Health Circular HC(80)8 outlines the provisions relating to these budgetary control arrangements. In particular DHAs should arrange their services into management units, each with an administrator and a director of nursing services. These would be directly accountable to the district administrator and district nursing officer respectively, and of appropriate seniority to discharge an individual responsibility in conjunction with a senior member of the medical staff. Within this structure, budgetary control and cash limit arrangements should provide for the maximum local delegation consistent with overall control of the DHA cash limit. District Treasurers should also provide financial advice, as necessary, to the budget-holder at unit level through improved financial information systems.

It is clear that budgetary control should not usually be operated on a district-wide functional basis but should operate at the unit level as follows:

(i)   Nursing budgets – responsibility of each unit's director of nursing services and ultimately the district nursing officer.
(ii) Hotel and support services – responsibility of each hospital administrator and ultimately the district administrator.
(iii) Clinical service budgets – local arrangements needed to decide whether budgets should be the responsibility of a district officer or a unit officer.

Below the UMG level the structure of budgets will vary enormously between DHAs. Take, for example, the nursing budget which in some DHAs might be broken down to senior nursing officer level while in other DHAs budgets might be given to each ward. Similar variations might be found in the treatment of paramedical service budgets. These budgets might be the responsibility of a district officer, as in Figure 10, or alternatively responsibility might be assigned to a UMG member or even the UMG as a whole.

The main rationale for the introduction of unit budgeting was the need to increase the speed of decision making in DHAs. Since budgets were to be delegated to the unit level, unit managers would be able to make quicker decisions without the need to refer to higher authority. Given the variation

Figure 10 – Outline of a Typical Structure for Unit Budgetary Control

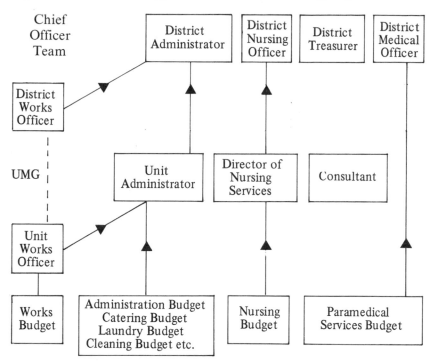

in practice of unit budgeting it would appear to be a difficult task to identify any improvement that has been achieved in the speed of decision making and we are not aware of any studies of this kind. Consequently we are forced to rely on some commonsense general principles which might help to ensure that unit budgeting contributed to quicker decision making. Two of these are discussed below:

a. *Delegation of Budgets*

As mentioned previously, below the UMG level the number and structure of budgets varies considerably between DHAs. However, bearing in mind the earlier comments about budgets being a form of delegated authority, it would seem desirable for budgets to be delegated to the lowest possible level. Consequently, it would be better to delegate the nursing budget down to ward level than to leave it at nursing officer (NO) level. Nevertheless, although this principle of maximum delegation is a good one it must be considered with care. Firstly, not everyone in the organisation has the managerial ability to be a budget holder and there is no point in delegating budgets to people who cannot adequately manage them. Secondly, the treasurers department might not have the resources to cope with the workload generated by a large number of budgets. Thirdly, the workload involved in managing a budget might adversely affect the time that some staff can contribute towards their main duty of patient care. Fourthly, delegating budgets downwards reduces the flexibility for the switching of resources.

b. Virement

Virement means the freedom to switch resources from one budget head to another budget. The scope of virement powers laid down in the DHAs standing financial instructions will determine the flexibility available to managers. For example, instead of having to obtain permission from higher authority, a unit administrator might have authority to vire resources between say the catering budget and the administration budget thus speeding up his response to a particular problem. Similarly the UMG might have the power to vire resources between say the nursing and works budgets for the unit. In this respect the unit administrator as the UMGs budget co-ordinator should make such virement quick to implement, provided that the financial implications have been assessed and agreed by the Treasurer beforehand.

However, the topic of virement must be treated with caution. The DHA on the advice of the DMT will have already agreed the authority's plans and detailed budgets. Too much freedom for UMGs to vire resources between budgets can easily lead to these plans and priorities being distorted. Thus a balance must be struck between the need for delegation and the need to ensure that objectives are attained.

8.3   Budgeting and Bugetary Control

As mentioned above, a budget is really a form of plan. More precisely, in the context of the NHS, a budget can be described as a statement, in financial terms, of existing activities of a health authority plus any proposed service changes during a year. This budget can be analysed between budget holders or a group of budget holders within that authority. It is clear therefore that a budget can only be prepared correctly after considering the planned acivities of each department, for the forthcoming year. When discussing planning in earlier chapters, we noted that for planning to be useful, annual programmes should be derived from the strategic plans. In a similar manner the budgets for a health authority and its departments should be derived from annual programmes. While this process should be followed completely it does not imply that all the proposals in an annual programme are automatically included in the budget. Ultimately, the authority must contain its expenditure within its cash limit. When a DHA is finally notified of its cash limit it is quite possible that it will not have sufficient funds to implement all aspects of the programme for that year and consequently, a choice must be made between priorities.

Another problem with health authority budgets is the existence of demand-based services. An example of this would be the catering budget, whereby all in-patients who come into hospital must be fed. Thus, if the number of in-patients admitted is greater than expected, it is quite common for the catering budget to be flexed to reflect the increased demand. The key question is how this increase in the catering budget is to be financed given the cash limit. In the context of a DHA we suggest that there are two main approaches:

a. Reserves

The District Treasurer might retain contingency reserves to enable him to finance any unforeseen items of expenditure. The danger with such reserves is that if no emergencies arise in the year, there tends to be a year end spending spree to avoid large under-spendings and to ensure that funds are not lost. We would not favour the use of reserves to meet such emergencies.

b. Prudent Financial Management

Sound financial management should require the Treasurer to arrange the DHAs financial affairs so that modest unforeseen items of expenditure can be financed in various ways. For example, underspending on departmental budgets may be reclaimed and used for additional spending by other departments – this principle of virement requires that the budgets are adjusted by a transfer of funds rather like the procedures outlined in Chapter 5, for transfers between capital and revenue.

8.4   Budget Preparation

Basically there are two approaches to preparing departmental budgets in an organisation:

a. The Incremental Approach

This approach to budget preparation takes as its starting point, the previous years budget. Thus the starting point for the 1984/85 budget will be the budget for 1983/84 which in turn will have been based on the 1982/83 budget and so on. Changes to the previous years budget will be made but, by and large, these will only be at the margin. Any incremental activities that the department has to undertake in the coming year might be reflected by an increased budget, and vice-versa for reduced activities. The bulk of the budget is however left unchallenged in that budget holders are not asked to justify each year the reasons for carrying out the various departmental activities and thus incurring expenditure. For example, each year, the portering budget for a hospital may be based on the assumption that internal mail needs to be distributed twice a day. Rarely is the question asked: *would daily deliveries be adequate?* If a single delivery would be satisfactory, the portering budget could be reduced and the resources released could be used elsewhere. Admittedly in this era of cut-backs these sorts of questions are being asked more frequently, but they should be asked at every opportunity if management is to ensure the best use of resources. Thus the main weakness of the traditional approach to budget preparation is that the bulk of an organisations expenditure is not challenged and any inefficiencies or mis-use of resources is perpetuated. To a large extent, budgeting in the NHS is based on this incremental approach whereby the budget for a year is really little more than a roll-forward from the previous year.

b. Zero Based Budgeting (ZBB)

In response to the deficiencies of the incremental approach to budget preparation, ZBB was developed, mainly in the USA. The main thrust of ZBB is that no part of a departmental budget is automatically carried forward to a future year without justification. In its pure form, ZBB required managers, each year, to attach not only a cost to each of the departments activities or planned activities, but also a valuation of the benefits accruing from that activity. All the activities of the organisation are then ranked in order of desirability, as measured by their net benefits, i.e. benefits minus costs. If a particular activity shows no net benefit to the organisation then of course, it would not be considered for implementation at all. Given that the organisation has limited resources, not all the activities will be capable of implementation and so a cut-off point must be drawn. All the activities above the cut-off point will be implemented or continued while all those below the line will either not be implemented or will be discontinued. In this way, top management ensures that every year full consideration is given to the way in which the organisation uses resources and ensures that only priorities are implemented.

Although, in theory, ZBB is highly desirable, in practice it has proved difficult to implement in its pure form, for the following reasons:

(i)   It is difficult to quantify and value the benefits arising from organisational activities.
(ii) Some services must be provided by statute even if a ZBB procedure finds them to be a low priority. For example, a ZBB procedure might find that monitoring of private nursing homes is not a priority but the service must still be provided.
(iii) It is not easy to discontinue certain activities even if they are of low priority. For example, manpower cannot be easily disposed of or redeployed. Contracts might have been taken out for the supply of materials and services and these cannot be terminated without a cost being incurred.
(iv) ZBB procedures are themselves time-consuming, bureaucratic and expensive to operate.

For these reasons ZBB has tended to fall out of fashion in recent years. However, most of the criticisms of ZBB apply to it in pure form and we believe that a less complex form of ZBB could still be usefully applied in DHA's. This less complex form can be termed priority base budgeting (PBB). The major criticism of ZBB was the difficulty and work involved in quantifying and valuing the benefits of departmental activities. PBB gets around this problem by only asking managers to rank the activities of their department or service in what they believe to be the priority order. For example, for the speech therapy service, the following ranking of activities might be decided upon by the senior speech therapist:

(1)   treatment of child stammerers
(2)   treatment of adults suffering from strokes
(3)   treatment of adult stammerers.

No attempt is made to quantify the net benefits of these services. Once such a ranking has been performed by all departments, for all activities, the details, together with the costs of implementing each item, would be submitted to the DMT. The DMT would then consider all the planned activities of all the departments and would recommend an order of priority to the DHA. Clearly, those departments activities with a high ranking would be likely to be implemented or continued but activities with a low ranking might be discontinued or rejected in favour of activities of another department. Thus, in the example, the treatment of adult stammerers could be discontinued or reduced in favour of a high priority from another different service such as improved obstetric services.

PBB is designed to encourage managers to examine their activities and to decide on priorities thus enabling top management to consider the activities of the organisation as a whole. Whether we use PBB or the incremental approach, whereby departmental activities are not really examined, it is desirable that the budget for a department or service is based on its planned work load. In the next seciton we shall discuss why this is not usually done by health authorities.

8.5   Inadequate Budget Base

If budgetary control is to be effective, it is essential that individual budgets realistically reflect the expected or planned workload of a department and that such budgets be perceived as being realistic by the relevant budget-holder. Many health authority budgets are in fact not related to the workload of a department or service. As mentioned previously, most budgets have been inherited from the past and the budget for the following year is usually based primarily on the current years budget with adjustments being made to reflect:

(a)   marginal changes in workload
(b)   pay and price increases.

Such a practice clearly means that in many cases departmental budgets are completely unrealistic and consequently the budget holder does not feel committed to achieving his particular budget. Having commented on the lack of workload related budgets, it is not so easy to develop a solution. There is a considerable lack of statistics about the workload of departments and services and the costs of performing a particular workload. Although these difficulties are accepted, we believe that progress can be made in a number of cases and that the development of workload-based budgets is one of the most desperately needed improvements in budgetary control in DHAs. Consider, for example, the following functions:

a.   Support and Technical Services

Under this heading we include such services as catering, cleaning, laundry, engineering maintenance and works maintenance. It is relatively easy in these cases to develop measures of workload. For example:

(i)   catering – number of meals prepared
(ii) cleaning – area cleaned.

Many DHAs do in fact utilise such measures in compiling budgets for these types of departments.

b. Para-Medical Services

In this group we include hospital departments such as pathology and radiography. The difficulty in preparing budgets for these departments is that the workload itself is extremely varied because of the different kinds of tests that are performed. To prepare budgets rationally for such departments it is necessary to know:

(i)   the number and type of tests to be performed
(ii) the workload involved in each type of test.

Statistics will usually be available about the numbers of different tests that have been performed in the previous year. An examination of the annual programme of the DHA should enable some sort of estimate to be prepared of how departmental workload will change in the ensuing year. For example, if it is planned to provide a further six gynaecology beds, it should be possible to assess the increased workload in terms of the number of tests to be performed. Thus we should be able to estimate the numbers and types of tests to be performed in the following year, but we then need to know the workload involved for each type of test.

We believe, however, that some progress can be made in developing workload measures, albeit in a somewhat subjective manner. To begin with the workload of the pathology departments can be classified by types of test. The next step would be to assess the average time spent on a particular kind of test, either by scientifically measuring the time spent performing a particular task, or by requesting the head of the department to give his assessment of the average time required. Once this has been done, the measures of time can easily be converted into unit costs for each test. For example, the labour element of unit costs themselves can be derived by using current pay rates for pathology technicians and calculating a labour cost per test.

The labour budget for the pathology department can therefore be derived by multiplying the forecast numbers of each type of test by the budgeted unit cost of that test and summating for all tests. We are not suggesting here that labour costs can be regarded as a marginal cost with the labour budget for pathology being flexed in response to changed levels of workload. It is quite possible that increased workload could be accommodated within the present departmental budget with no additional labour being required. What this approach does do, is give some idea of what should be the pathology labour budget for a planned level of workload. A similar exercise could be performed for non-pay costs by multiplying the forecast numbers of tests by a pre-determined estimated usage of materials per test. Adding together labour costs, materials costs and managerial costs would then give a total budget for the pathology department based on a forecast workload and would not be merely the rolling forward of the previous years budget. If the department maintains at some future date that their estimates of workload per test are no longer relevant, because of such factors as technological change, then adjustments might be made, but only after a thorough review has been carried out. We believe that such an approach to budget preparation would be a great improvement on the usual approach of merely rolling forward the previous year's budget.

c. Direct Patient Care Services

The major item under this heading would be nursing and in fact nursing comprises approximately one third of health authority costs. Unfortunately, at present there appears to be very little in the way of workload measures for nursing services that would enable one to compute the level of nursing required for a particular number of patients. The main potential would seem to arise from studies of nurse dependency of patients. These might provide some local information which could be used for the preparation of nurse budgets. Such dependency studies would indicate the different workloads that would arise for wards caring for various types of patients.

8.6   Responsibility and Incomplete Budgets

A key feature of any system of budgetary control is the concept of responsibility accounting. By this we mean that in any organisation, if expenditure is to be adequately controlled, it is desirable that the following conditions have been met:

(a) all components of the organisation's expenditure are made the responsibility of some individual.

(b) individuals are only held responsible for those items of expenditure over which they can actually exert control.

Failure to meet the first condition means that there are some items of expenditure at a 'loose-end' with no one assigned to control them. Failure to meet the second condition reduces the effectiveness and reliability of the budgetary control system.

This idea of responsibility is an ideal which will not be totally achieved in any organisation. A particular difficulty in a DHA concerns the drugs budget. Frequently it is the case that the pharmacist is designated the budget holder for drugs and is nominally held responsible for drugs expenditure. However, the level of expenditure on drugs is almost completely determined by the clinician who is not usually designated a budget holder.

Another case where responsibility accounting is breached concerns incomplete budgets. Take for example the catering budget. The catering budget will include staff costs, provisions, but will not usually include an amount for energy costs. The energy budget would be held by a works officer. However, the actual consumption of energy in the catering department would be determined by the catering staff and not by the works officer, thus reducing the effectiveness of budgetary control. Many other examples of this type can be quoted.

8.7   Participation in Budget Preparation

For motivational reasons, it is usually thought to be good practice that budget holders should actively participate in the budget-setting procedures of their departments and that budgets should not merely be passed down from higher authority. By being involved and agreeing to specific targets, the budget holder is thought to commit himself to his budget and will therefore strive harder to meet it than if it had just been imposed.

Some studies have, in fact, suggested that in health authorities, budget holders do not actively participate in the preparation of either pay or non-pay budgets for their departments and that most budget work is performed in the Treasurers department. There may be many reasons for this lack of a true participative approach as opposed to a pseudo-participative approach involving cursory consultation. We suggest the following, in order of importance, as being the main reasons for the lack of participative approach:

(a) an absence of workload measures for budget preparation
(b) budget holders being too concerned with their professional work to be involved with budget setting
(c) budget holders not being really competent in financial matters
(d) the rigidity of NHS funding arrangements.

8.8   Reporting Systems

For budgetary control to be effective, it is essential that an adequate reporting system exists to convey information, to budget holders, about their budgetary performance over a period of time, usually a month. The key features of a reporting system appear to be the following:

(a)   Timeliness – budgetary control reports should be received by budget holders, very soon after the end of the month.
(b)   Content – reports should be comprehensive for budget holders to exercise effective control.
(c)   Advice – finance staff should provide adequate assistance and support to budget holders to assist them in interpreting and acting on their reports.

Historically, it appears that budgetary control in health authorities has been unsatisfactory as far as timeliness is concerned. Surveys have been produced[3] showing that budget holders have sometimes had to wait up to six weeks adter the end of the month before receiving their budgetary control statements. Although the situation may have improved in recent years, we feel that in many authorities, budget holders are not getting information quickly enough for control to be effective. The two main reasons for this appear to be:

a.   Inadequate Computer Systems

Although the introduction of the Standard Accounting System (SAS) and subsequent technological developments improved the quality of budgetary control in some health authorities, we believe that health authorities are still too involved with processing on large regional mainframe computers. Such a method of operating budgetary control creates an inherent delay in the production of budgetary control information and we would prefer to see much greater development of on-line budgetary control systems on smaller computers at the DHA level. Only in this way will budget holders obtain a really fast service.

b.   Obsession with Detail

In many health authorities it appears that budgetary control reports may be delayed by up to a week to enable finance staff to amend them manually for greater accuracy, for example by including creditors. Ideally, perhaps the best solution to this could be the introduction of a comprehensive commitment accounting system. Failing that we believe it best that information should be despatched as quickly as possible even if it is not totally accurate. Consideration might in fact be given to the operation of budgetary control on a cash payment basis since such an approach appears to provide very quick information.

As far as content is concerned, we believe the two most important features here are:

(a) the degree of flexibility in report designs
(b) the provision of non-financial data.

A recent publication has explained that for budgetary control to be effective, budget holders should be consulted about the design of their reports and given a chance to state what they require. To achieve this, a reporting system with sufficient flexibility in report design is needed. It will suffice to say that in the NHS the Standard Accounting System does provide flexibility in report designs.

Some budget holders would find it useful if reports also contained non-financial information. Information could be provided about the resource inputs of a department such as the number of man hours worked in a month. Alternatively, information could be shown about the work actually performed. by a department in the period and as examples we suggest the following:

(a) Pathology   - numbers of tests perhaps classified by type
(b) Catering   - numbers of meals
(c) Operating Theatres - numbers of operations classified by type.

We believe it is important that this kind of information be incorporated on budgetary control reports, for without it, such reports merely show what a department has spent and not what it has achieved in a period. Furthermore, this activity data could be linked with the financial data to provide unit cost information such as cost per pathology test. This is one facet of budgetary control where health authorities have not advanced as far as other parts of the public sector.

Finally we come to the need for finance department support for budget holders. It is sometimes said that the good management accountant spends most of his time out of the office and although this might be extreme we believe it contains some truth. Most budget holders in a health authority are not financially trained and are perhaps not totally competent in financial matters. Consequently there is a need for finance staff to visit budget holders regularly to discuss their budgets and to offer advice about aspects of budgetary control.

8.9 Developments in Budgetary Control

In a book of this nature, it is difficult to summarise in any great detail all possible developments that are taking place in the NHS with budgetary control systems. However, in this section we have discussed briefly two classes of development which are taking place:

(a) Clinical involvement in budgetary control
(b) Improved reporting systems.

The first of these has some far reaching implications on the behavioural and ethical front while the second is merely a set of technical improvements to the present structure of budgetary control.

a. Clinical Involvement in Budgetary Control

We have already briefly discussed the problem of the breakdown of responsibility accounting in budgetary control resulting from the power of the clinicians to influence levels of expenditure. It is often held that the consultant and his medical team's activity can exert considerable influence over levels of expenditure. We believe that this clinical power is over-exaggerated and in reality is restricted to a relatively minor influence on levels of expenditure. Clinicians can make decisions that will affect expenditure on relatively few items, i.e. drugs, which comprise only a very small percentage of a DHAs expenditure. One point that is clear is that DHAs spend about 75% of the revenue on manpower and such expenditure is not directly influenced by clinicians. Similarly, other items such as energy and hotel costs are also not under the clinicians influence. They do have a somewhat greater influence over the workload of the hospital and its various classes of staff. For example, clinical decisions about patients will affect the workload of nursing staff. However, such influences only have marginal effects on levels of expenditure but do affect the efficiency with which resources are used.

To our knowledge the influence of clinicians on the commitment of resources is not known precisely as evidence is not available as to the actual structure of clinical decision making, namely what decisions do doctors take and what decisions are taken by other staff such as nurses.

Following on from the above, the question usually asked is: *if clinicians have such influence over the efficient use of resources, why not involve them in the budgetary control process?* On the face of it, this seems a simple solution; budgets could be prepared for individual clinicians or groups of clinicians and some form of control exercised over these budgets.

It is not intended that such 'specialty budgets' replace unit budgets as these will still be required, to ensure that the DHA's spending is contained within its cash limit. The main advantage of specialty budgets is in helping to control the longer term pattern of resource usage in the DHA.

Several experiments are being or have been conducted into the involvement of clinicians in the budgeting process, and we have identified three of these:

(i)   St. Thomas's Hospital Experiments
(ii) Clinical Accountability Service Planning and Evaluation (CASPE) experiments
(iii) NHS Management Inquiry: Management Budgets

These are discussed briefly below:

i. St. Thomas's Hospital The basis of the St. Thomas's approach is that the functional budgets of the district were reclassified along specialty lines. For example the radiography budget would be analysed over medical specialties according to the planned usage by each of those specialties. Once all functional budgets have been analysed over specialities, a total specialty budget can be obtained based on the planned activity of each specialty over the coming year.

Once these budgets have been prepared, the monitoring system operates throughout the year. Actual expenditure is reclassified over specialties on the same basis used to prepare the specialty budgets.

Comparisons of specialty costs against specialty budgets are made and management reports are prepared showing:

(i)   variances due to actual clinical activity differing from budgeted activity
(ii) other variances such as over/under spending.

Although control over specialty budgets would not be as strictly applied as for functional budgets, clinicians would be involved in decisions about correcting any variances of specialty cost from budget. This might be regarded as a loose form of control over the allocation of the resources involving clinicians, rather than the tight form of functional or unit budgetary control which tends to exclude clinicians.

ii. CASPE Experiments This project is being undertaken at several locations under the aegis of the King Edward's Hospital Fund.

At the heart of the CASPE approach are a series of planning agreements with clinical teams (PACTs) and these agreements will cover:

planned workload of the team, resources required, planned achievements etc. During the course of the year, it is then necessary to feedback information about activity and costs, to the clinical team so that actual performance may be compared with what is contained in the PACT. Any deviations from plan may require changes, either by revising unrealistic plans or by changes in clinical practice and/or activity. These changes might sometimes involve expenditure but other times will involve changes in admission, discharge and investigative procedures. Therefore this approach is more than just a narrow budgetary control system.

iii. NHS Management Inquiry : Management Budgets The NHS Management Inquiry (The Griffiths Report) commissioned a series of projects into management budgeting in four DHAs, the aim being to develop a system of budgeting/budgetary control involving clinicians as budget holders. The development work is being carried out by two firms of management consultants: Coopers and Lybrand Associates and Arthur Young McClelland Moore. Each firm of consultants is involved with two DHAs each.

It is beyond the scope of this book to fully describe the management budgeting approach. It will suffice to say here that management budgeting attempts to simultaneously overcome four main problems: the lack of involvement of clinicians; the breach of responsibility accounting; incremental budget-setting; and poor quality management information.

Although few could object to such development projects being undertaken, we are not certain yet what problems will be encountered. For example, clinicians are not trained in aspects of management and neither is managerial expertise regarded as essential or desirable for promotion. We believe such approaches will only be completely successful when future generations of clinicians have been trained in aspects of management as well as the conventional subjects taught at medical school. We would ask the following questions about specialty budgeting and related activities:

(i) *Would clinicians be willing to become involved in the process of setting budgets and controlling expenditure?* There is some evidence that many will not.

(ii) Even if they were willing, *would clinicians be effective in dealing with budgeting matters, given their general lack of managerial and financial experience?* Doctors are trained primarily as doctors and not as managers. This objection, however, could also be levied at nurses and para-medical staff who in fact have gained an understanding and experience of budgetary control in recent years.

(iii) *Is it ethically correct for clinicians to be involved in these matters given that their primary responsibility is to the individual patient? Who among us wishes to have his or her treatment prescribed by a doctor with one eye on his budget?* However, one must always bear in mind the idea of opportunity costs. Every extra pound spent by Doctor A means somebody, somewhere else, has to spend less since resources available to a DHA are finite. As well as considering the patients currently under his care, the doctor needs to consider those patients awaiting care.

(iv) *On what information base would specialty budgets be prepared? In how much detail would they be prepared? Would they be flexible budgets? How strictly or loosely would specialty budgetary control be operated – if strictly, would clinicians accept it and if loosely, is it of any use?*

(v) If clinicians are to be held accountable for the expenditure of their specialties, we must be able to attribute items of expenditure to them. This form of specialty costing would need to be more accurate than specialty costing for planning purposes. *Are the required costing techniques available?*

As we have already said, we believe that clinicians have little influence on the level of most items of NHS expenditure. We believe that much of the thrust of clinical budgeting is misdirected. What clinicians undoubtedly have influence over is the way in which resources are used to treat patients. Thus they have control over:

(a) the number of patients treated
(b) the type of patient treated
(c) the way in which that patient is treated.

Consequently, we believe the emphasis should be placed on the setting of performance and treatment objectives at specialty level and the feedback of information on clinical performance by means of a set of performance measures. The use of such an approach might influence clinical behaviour. The management budgeting approach described above points to this.

b. Improved Reporting Systems

Given the alleged limitations of the Standard Accounting System mentioned in Section 8.8, it is interesting to note the latest development being undertaken in the NHS. It is the Interactive Resource Information System (IRIS). This system, which is being developed at the West Midlands RHA, is really a modern SAS and aims to retain the best features of SAS while adding on enhancements such as on-line interrogation of files and a better interface with other information systems. At the time of writing it is too early to comment on the merits of such a development.

What we have discussed above is a development taking place within the NHS. At this point in time it is appropriate to say a word about the financing of computing services in the NHS. Traditionally, RHAs have provided a free computing service to DHAs in that no charge was made to DHAs for the use made of RHA computing services although clearly every extra £ spent by the RHA implies a £ less for DHA patient services. Recently, moves have been made to place computing serivces on a more commercial basis whereby the RHAs would charge their DHAs according to the use made of such services. Given the Government's policy of competitive tendering for support services, the next step must be for DHAs to consider the RHA computer service as one of a number of organisations capable of providing computing services. There will be many private sector computing organisations eager to enter such a large market and RHA computer centres will need to become far more commercially and customer orientated.

8.10   Unit Costing in the NHS

We have already discussed in Chapter 7 the problems of actually measuring the output of health services. As a consequence of our inability to measure output and hence the effectiveness of health services it is not really possible to measure the efficiency of services. Unit costs are often put forward as possible measures of efficiency; for example, if the cost per patient/day of running hospital A is 10% higher than the cost in hospital B the latter is often alleged to be more efficient than the former. The point of course is that such information says nothing about the quality of service provided in these hospitals. Hospital A could be more expensive because it gives a better quality and more appropriate service.

In spite of their limitations, we believe that unit costing data can be a useful component of financial control in the following ways:

(i)   Some activities of DHAs can be physically measured and so unit cost data can provide useful measures of efficiency. For example cost per mile run of the ambulance service might indicate the efficiency of one authority compared with another.

(ii) Unit cost information can indicate those activities requiring further investigations. For example, if we compare the costs of treating patients in one hospital with those in another, then any cost differences provide the basis for further investigation. Too often cost differences are glibly explained away in terms of better or worse standards of service without this explanation ever being investigated let alone verified. used in this way, unit cost data merely acts as a pointer to more detailed studies.

An important point about the use of unit cost data in measuring efficiency is that unit costs would primarily be used in a comparative manner. Unit costs can be compared in the following ways:

(i)   Inter-Authority- unit costs of one DHA can be compared with those of others or the average of others both within and outside the region.

(ii) Intra-Authority – the unit costs of one hospital in the DHA can be compared with other hospitals in the same DHA.

(iii) Inter-temporal – unit costs can be compared over time. After removing the effects of inflation by means of indices we can see if unit costs have changed in real terms over a period of time.

If unit costs are to be useful, it is essential that as far as possible we compare like with like. Thus it is necessary that the units used are the same and that the costs included are the same. Also we must compare like activities. It is no use comparing the unit costs of an acute care hospital with those of a geriatric hospital – they are too different in nature. As far as actual practice is concerned, the NHS, as with other parts of the public sector, abounds with unit costs data. These may be produced by the DHA, the RHA or the DHSS but in the main they can be grouped as follows:

(a)   Support service unit costs – such unit costs as cost per meal, cost per square foot of domestic services.

(b)   Hospital costs – unit costs of treating patients may be produced for individual hospitals, such as cost per case or cost per patient/day.

(c)   Specialty costs – in other chapters we have already discussed the use of specialty costs within the authority for RAWP purposes and planning purposes respectively. If such specialty costs become readily available then clearly they could be used by DHAs in a comparative manner. More specifically, we believe that such comparisons could be made in two different ways by two different groups of people:

    (i)   Monitoring by DHA – each DHA could compare its cost per patient for a particular specialty with the corresponding cost for other DHAs. Clearly such comparisons will say nothing about the quality of service provided but will provide the basis for future investigations. However, evidence exists to suggest that specialties themselves are not homogeneous in nature and one specialty might incorporate many diverse activities with differing costs. Thus even comparisons of specialty costs might be too broad and

comparisons should be made at a lower level, such as disease costs or patient costs.

(ii) *Self-monitoring by clinicians* – It seems to us that progress could be made by presenting clinicians with information about the financial consequences of their clinical decisions. By doing this, one hopes to influence their behaviour rather than attempting the somewhat oppressive approach of imposing budgets on them. Consequently clinicians could be presented with unit costs, over a period, for their particular specialty compared with comparative unit costs for similar hospitals. Although many people are sceptical about the reaction of clinicians to such information we feel that such experiments might prove worthwhile.

In Chapter 7, we discussed the topic of patient costing systems. As with planning, we believe such systems would be more flexible than specialty costing systems and the following kinds of unit cost comparisons could be made:

(i)   Comparisons of treating diseases.
(ii) Comparisons of clinicians within the same specialty.
(iii) Comparisons of wards.

The main advantage of patient costing is its accounting basis. In principle, it adopts the approach of job costing, and as in an industrial setting, can provide a powerful management tool for DHAs in both controlling and planning specific services and specialties.

8.11   Internal Audit

In any organisation of a reasonable size, internal audit is regarded as an essential instrument of financial control. Although DHAs will be subject to an annual external audit, this is not a continuous examination of its activities and is, therefore, bound to be somewhat limited in depth. However, DHAs will wish to be assured that systems of financial control are satisfactory at all times, and to this end the organisation would employ an internal audit section whose tasks would include the following:

(a) Assessment of the strengths and weaknesses of systems of financial control;

(b) Prevention and detection of fraud;

(c) Detection of waste and inefficiency.

It will be noticed that the tasks of the internal auditor are similar to those of the external auditor discussed in Chapter 5. The key difference however is that since the internal auditor is a full-time employee of the organisation, he will be able to examine issues in much greater depth than the external auditor would ever be able to do.

Prior to the 1984 reorganisation, internal audit was a poor relation in the NHS. Audit sections were usually understaffed and in some cases non-existent. Given the importance now attached to internal audit we can only wonder how adequate at that time, were the broader aspects of financial control such as the security of financial systems. The 1982 reorganisation placed much more emphasis on internal audit. The responsibility for the task throughout DHA was placed squarely on the shoulders of the Treasurer. Similarly, the internal audit of RHA activities was the responsibility of the Regional Treasurer.

As a result of this 'recognition' of internal audit, staff was appointed in all health authorities and headed by a Chief Internal Auditor. In spite of this improvement in the status of internal audit, several reports suggested that there were still considerable weaknesses in internal audit. Some of these are discussed here:

a. Staffing

Some years ago a report suggested that the staffing of internal audit departments was inadequate, in terms of quantity and quality, for audit duties to be carried out satisfactorily. Many internal audit departments did not have sufficient staff resources to carry out basic financial systems audit let alone the more modern value-for-money or cost effectiveness types of audit. We are not convinced that this situation has changed greatly.

Too often, audit is seen as the poor relation of finance departments and audit staff often complain of the inadequate remuneration and promotion prospects vis-a-vis other finance posts. Although this may be the case, it is easy to see that when health authorities are experiencing limited growth or even cutbacks in resources, requests for an additional internal auditor will have to compete with demands such as additional doctors, nurses and medical equipment. In this situation internal audit will seldom be seen as a priority.

b. Computer Audit:

In most health authorities today, the computer is a key component in any system of financial administration. Computers are used routinely in such activities as payroll preparation, payments to creditors and budgetary control. The growth in the use of computers for financial services has led to the development of computer audit. As this is not a book on computer audit, we have not described in detail its nature, but in summary it includes the following:

(i)   *Design work* – computer auditors will be consulted about the design of computer systems to ensure that adequate checks and balances are built into the system. Also the auditors will wish to ensure that adequate audit trails exist so that transactions can be followed through the system.

(ii) *Operational aspects* – the auditor will conduct regular examinations to ensure computer-based systems are operating in a satisfactory manner. He will be concerned to ensure that the inputs into the systems such as creditor invoices, match up with the outputs, such as cheques drawn. He will also wish to ensure that the various control procedures that were laid down are actually being followed.

(iii) *File interrogation* – the auditor will periodically test the adequacy of systems of financial control by interrogating the computer files using special interrogation programs. Thus he might request details of any salary payments over say £1000 per month to check for any possible frauds involving the payment of salaries and wages.

In DHAs, computer audit is a relatively undeveloped subject and there are clearly weaknesses in the approach of internal and also external audit. Furthermore the problems of computer audit are compounded by the structure of computing in the NHS. The usual computing arrangements are that computing services are provided by the RHA on its mainframe machine, on behalf of the DHAs. Now, although the financial activities of the DHA are dealt with on the RHA computer, it is still the District Treasurer who is responsible to his DHA for financial control of systems in the authority. Consequently many District Treasurers may object to a computer auditor employed by the RHA carrying out computer audit on their behalf.

Although the RHA's internal auditor would be able to perform some audit work on matters such as control procedures and program verification, he would not have access to DHA computer files for interrogation purposes. The corollary to this is that because of their size, most DHAs are unlikely to be able to employ a specialist computer auditor of their own. Although there is no real solution to the problem, it appears to us that a reasonable compromise can be found either by allowing regionally based computer auditors to have access to DHA files under the supervision of the District Treasurer, or for two or more DHAs to join forces and appoint a joint specialist in computer audit.

c. Capital Audit

Health authorities are continually involved in a variety of capital projects such as the construction of hospitals and health centres, enlargement of present hospitals and renovation work. Because of the large sums of money involved there is a key role here for the internal auditor. The audit of capital projects can be divided into three categories:

(i) *Prior to construction* – the internal auditor can perform such tasks as assessment of the financial stability of potential contractors, examination of proposed schemes.

(ii) *During construction* – the internal auditor will be concerned with ensuring that proper records are kept dealing with matters such as payments to contractors and the proper control of variation orders.

(iii) *After construction* – the internal auditor will wish to be satisfied that the contractor's final account is correct. As well as arithmetic checking, he will be concerned to ensure that the organisation receives what it has paid for and that contractors have not failed to meet the specifications. He may also be concerned with such things as the standard of workmanship and the quality of materials used. These latter tasks may be regarded as the value-for-money kind of audit. In conducting such audits, the auditor may run into some conflict with other professionals such as quantity surveyors but we believe he should persevere and not let professional jargon and pride divert him from his tasks.

It has been suggested that the capital audit performed by health authories is mainly restricted to the first two categories. Although internal auditors check final accounts for accuracy they have little involvement in any of the value-for-money style audits. This seems rather disturbing considering that a new hospital can cost up to £30 million to build and a new health centre can easily exceed £½ million. If we were considering such sums of revenue money it is unlikely that health authorities would spend that amount without verifying that they had received what they paid for.

These deficiencies in capital audit can be accounted for by two main causes:

(i)   As mentioned earlier, most internal audit sections have insufficient staff to allow one member to concentrate on capital project audit.
(ii) Auditors are usually financially trained and have no experience of the technical aspects of building projects.

In spite of these problems, some authorities, however, do attempt this kind of post-completion audit by utilising the services of technical specialists, such as building officers, employed by the authority. While this is not the perfect solution it is clearly better than doing nothing. Generally, internal audit is still not given adequate emphasis and recognition by DHAs. Unfortunately, we do not see any change in this attitude in the near future.

d. The Salmon Report

In January 1983 the report of the DHSS/NHS Audit Working Group (the Salmon Report) was published.

The main conclusions of the report with regard to internal audit can be summarised as follows:

(i)   There should be an audit plan designed to achieve a minimum level of audit in all key areas of financial responsibility;
(ii) Consortia arrangements should be considered especially by the smaller DHAs;
(iii) Internal audit should be regarded as a training ground for all finance staff.
(iv) Internal audit should include a review of management systems to secure value-for-money.

In our opinion the Salmon Report is a rather disappointing report containing some rather unrealistic recommendations. Although the use of the audit plan to achieve a minimum acceptable level of audit is clearly the rational way to proceed, it is not necessarily a realistic approach. DHAs faced with tight management cost ceilings, staff reductions and cash limit squeezes are unlikely to want to proceed in this way. They are more likely to take a pragmatic line and decide on the amount of resources they can afford to deploy into audit rather than the amount the audit plan says they should deploy. This after all is the way in which decisions about the resources going to patient services are made.

e.   Value for Money (VFM) Audit

The term VFM audit has become popular parlance in recent years although it is really not a new idea. Furthermore, there appears to be considerable confusion as to what VFM audit actually is or even whether VFM studies should really be a part of audit at all. In Chapter 10 we have discussed in detail the nature and application of VFM studies in the NHS but in this section we restrict ourselves to a discussion of the role of audit in VFM studies. We believe that value for money can be considered in two parts:

(i)   The creation and utilisation of systems and procedures that will assist in the search for value or money;

(ii) An examination of the above systems with the aim of ensuring that they are being utilised adequately and that they continue to be effective.

In DHAs, based on the lessons of HC(80)8, we believe it is the role of UMGs to lead the search for value for money. To do this the UMG may need to create and utilise a variety of systems both formal and informal. It would not be the role of internal audit to interfere directly in the task of searching for better value for money. However, it would be the role of internal audit to ensure that the UMGs were actually making a positive attempt to search for value for money. Thus internal audit would need to examine the use of such systems. As an example of this we refer back to the discussion of investment appraisal in section 7.9. Such a systematic approach should be followed by UMGs to make the best use of scarce resources. It would not be appropriate for internal audit to comment on the priorities of the UMG derived from the system but it would be the job of internal audit to ensure that the UMGs did follow the correct approach of consultation, documentation etc.

Finally, although no one could be against the involvement of internal audit in the search for VFM as outlined above, we must refer back to the staffing problems discussed earlier. It appears to us that there are considerable weaknesses in conventional financing and compliance audit to be overcome before branching out into the realm of VFM audit.

9

Alternative Sources of Finance

9.1 Introduction

During 1983, great controversy arose over a 'leaked' secret report of the Government's Central Policy Review Staff (CPRS) – *The Think Tank* – concerning the long term financing of certain public services including the NHS. What this report did was highlight the dilemma that faces the NHS. The originators of the NHS believed that if sufficient resources were committed to the health services, eventually the demand for those services would be satisfied. In hindsight we know this view to be incorrect.

Figure 11 – Dilemma of NHS Finance

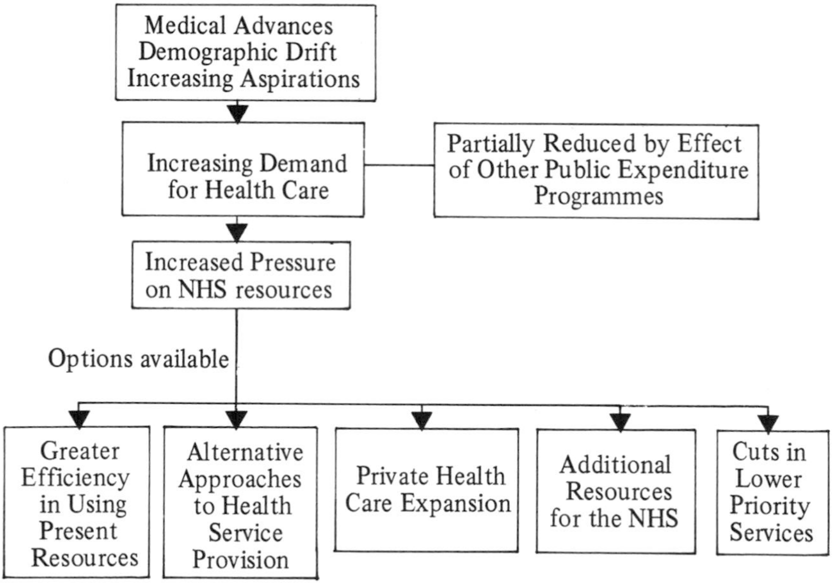

Advances in medical techniques have in themselves created the demand for a service where none previously existed. An obvious example of this phenomenom is the demand for articifial joint operations. Thirty years ago the surgical techniques were not developed and so the demand for this form of treatment was nil although the need remained unfulfilled. Today the technique is virtually commonplace and thus we have a demand for a service where none previously existed.

Nor are medical advances the only cause of increasing demand for health services. The growth in the numbers of the elderly in the population (demographic drift) also puts an increasing strain on the NHS as do the generally increasing aspiration levels of the population. All of these factors combine to pose a dilemma as to how the NHS should be financed in the longer term. The position is summarised in Figure 11.

What is shown above is that the increasing demand for health services could be met in a number of ways. Firstly it could be alleviated from outside the NHS itself by means of increased expenditure on other public expenditure programmes. Perhaps the most oft-quoted example concerns housing, where it is argued that increased housing investment would lead to better housing standards with a consequent reduction in certain illnesses and hence the need for health services.

In spite of these arguments we feel it unlikely that all the increases in demand for health care can be met from outside the NHS. It seems likely that the trend will be one of increasing pressure on the resources of the NHS and hence one needs to look for ways of alleviating this pressure. It appears to us that there are four main options available which can be mixed in various combinations as it is probable that they will all be applied to some degree or another. Let us briefly examine the options available.

a. Greater Efficiency

The increasing demand for health services could be met, at least partially, by the NHS using its present resources in a more efficient manner. The topics of efficiency and value-for-money have become increasingly important in recent years, in all parts of the public sector including the NHS. However it is important that improved efficiency is not a disguise for genuine cuts in the standards of service but reflects a real redeployment of resources.

The topic of improved efficiency is discussed in greater detail in Chapter 10.

b. Alternative Approaches

Another option might be to change the way in which health services are being provided, the aim being to meet existing future needs in a different way. One example might be to put more emphasis on preventative health care in the hope that in the longer term this would reduce the need for health care. Another alternative might be to provide a different pattern of health care by placing more emphasis on community care and less on hospital care on the assumption that community care is cheaper.

It is beyond the scope of this book to discuss this topic in any depth and the interested reader is referred elsewhere.

c. Private Health Care

Yet another way of reducing the pressure on the NHS might be to shift part of the burden on to the private health sector. It is unlikely that the private sector would be interested in providing some services such as those for mentally-handicapped and hence the issue largely concerns shifting part of the acute services to the private sector.

d. Additional Resources

Irrespective of what is done with the three previous options it seems likely to us that to ease the pressure on the NHS it will be necessary to provide at least some additional resources. This point is already recognised in the present method of financing by means of health authorities development additions. This can be used to cover the efects of demographic drift and improved medical technology. The outlook for future increases is outlined in Chapter 2. However, if additional resources are to be committed to the NHS it appears that this could be done either within the present financing structure or by the use of alternative and/or supplementary sources of finance.

The issues surrounding the possibility of alternative ways of financing the NHS will form the remainder of this chapter.

e. Cuts in Lower Priority Services

Finally, for the sake of completeness, we must make the point that if none of the four options were implemented the only possible outcome would be cuts in lower priority services in order to release resources for services related to the three factors of medical technology, demographic drift and increasing aspirations. Such cuts might be thinly spread across most NHS services or alternatively a more radical approach could be adopted by cutting out complete services.

9.2 Summary of the Present NHS Financing Method

Before commencing a discussion about alternative ways of financing the NHS, it might be valuable as a reminder to restate some of the main principles of the present method of finance.

The overall level of spending on the NHS is determined by the Government using the PESC methodology together with the Parliamentary Estimates. This is financed from three sources:

(a) charges, which account for about 3% of NHS finance
(b) a contribution from the National Insurance Fund which provides about 11%
(c) general taxation provides the balance of some 86%.

Charges are a limited source of finance and apply to items such as prescriptions, spectacles and dentistry. Their contribution is so small and specific that they can be disregarded as a significant source of finance in the present system. The second element, the National Insurance Fund, is also a specific contribution, but it is fashionable to consider that national insurance contributions are an element and extension of general taxation. For example, the effect of changes in national insurance are reflected in the Government's Retail Prices and Tax Index along with changes in taxes such as income tax and VAT. In this sense, the contribution from the National Insurance Fund can be combined with the contribution from general taxation.

Overall, we consider that the NHS can be seen as being financed almost entirely from general taxation. Patients are not required to pay directly for most services that they use. Because the services are already paid for, patients tend to see health services as free at the point of use. In these circumstances, the long term demand for health services is extremely large, possibly approaching infinity. Without a price mechanism to allow this demand to interact with the supply of health services, supply has to be determined by rationing. This results in the waiting list for services, so that patients are effectively held in a queue for the service that each requires.

It is probably this aspect of the present arrangements that evokes most hostility. Waiting lists are often seen as an indication of the inadequacy of health services, particularly their lack of flexibility and responsiveness to changes in the community's needs.

To alleviate these problems additional resources could be provided within the present financing structure. This could be achieved in a number of ways:

a. Economic Growth

If improvements in economic growth were to be achieved it would be possible for the NHS to have additional funds without the need for it to consume a greater proportion of the nations GDP. Although we have little detailed knowledge of macro economics it does not seem to us that this is a reasonable possibility. The Chancellor of the Exchequer's Autumn 1983 Economic Statement put public expenditure at 42% of GDP. If this percentage remains stable then increases in GDP should result in increases, in public expenditure, with the action of directing some of that increase into the NHS.

b. Transfers from Other Public Services

The Government could decide to provide additional funds for the NHS by cutting back on other public expenditure programmes thereby releasing funds which could be absorbed by the NHS. For this to be done would require the Government to alter its priorities for public expenditure programmes.

c. Increased Taxation or Borrowing

If neither of the above options is thought feasible or desirable then additional funds for the NHS could only come about as a result of increased taxation or extra Government borrowing. It is beyond the scope of this book to discuss the desirability of either of these options.

The alternative approach is to consider different ways in which the NHS might be financed and it is to this we now turn.

9.3   Alternative Methods of Finance

During 1982 the Government established a working party to consider alternative sources of finance for the NHS. Its members included civil servants and consultants with experience of the private sector. The general aim was to provide an assessment of alternatives available. Following completion of the report the Secretary of State announced to Parliament that the Government had no plans to change the present system of financing the NHS largely from taxation.

Hence it might be thought that the topic of alternative financing is now dead. We, however, feel that this should not be the case and we see it as quite conceivable that because of increasing demand for health services the issue should be revived soon. Consequently we believe it important to describe the alternatives most commonly put forward.

Before embarking on this description, it is important to recognise two features of the finance of the NHS. Firstly, the method of financing health services is often seen by some as being inextricably linked to political views. We do not believe that such an inevitable and permanent relationship exists, and we have considered the various alternatives on their financial merit. The second matter is that the method of finance is directly related to the provision and management of health services. In assessing the alternatives, we have also acknowledged their managerial implications.

The present method of finance has been criticised in two main respects. One is that the method of finance is totally inappropriate, and should be replaced. The second is that the existing method could be improved or enhanced and merely needs to be updated to reflect the current relative affluence of the community. In response to these criticisms, we have outlined three alternatives in this chapter. They are:

(a) Insurance Schemes
(b) Partial Charging
(c) Supplementary Income.

9.4 Insurance Schemes

Charging for health services is often advocated as an alternative method of finance. It is inconceivable that such an approach would be considered without some kind of insurance scheme. For example, treatment costs can be extremely high, sometimes as much as £20,000, and it is unlikely that most individuals could finance such a bill without the equalising effect of insurance cover. Three main types of insurance could be envisaged:

(a) wholly private and voluntary
(b) wholly public and compulsory
(c) a mix of these two.

a. Wholly Private and Voluntary

Private and voluntary insurance cover is similar to the method used in the USA. It could result in four categories of patients, those who:

(i) would be fully insured for any eventuality;

(ii) would be partly insured, and decide on how to deal with any further cost by either paying from his own resources or not availaing himself of the facilities;

(iii) would choose to pay all his health bills without resort to health insurance;

(iv) would choose not to seek the benefits of the health service because he would not be able to pay the premiums.

Clearly, an important aspect of such insurance cover is the creation of classes of patients that would be unable to have or afford access to health services.

The vision of individuals turning up at hospital only to be turned away because of a lack of financial standing may be largely unacceptable to many. Such a proposal may therefore be rejected as inappropriate.

A further implication of such a proposal is that while insurance cover would be available to meet the costs of acute and general treatment, it is unlikely to be available for such services as those for the mentally handicapped and the elderly. Consequently, the 'cinderella-type' services would continue to be financed from the public purse.

Private and voluntary health insurance does not automatically imply either private or public provision of health services. However, we believe that such a method is conducive to an expansion of private medical care. Should this link with private health care materialise, then its protagonists would probably claim that private treatment would result in a reduction in waiting time and more attention being given to each patient. While this may be true for a limited private health service, it would be important to establish the position if the whole population chose to classify themselves as (i) previously, namely to be insured for any eventuality. It is difficult to envisage all patients receiving earlier and better treatment without an increase in facilities because the number and type of patients would correspond with those who currently present themselves for treatment by the NHS. Merely changing the method of finance would not result in an improved service if all patients availed themselves of the same facilities.

The main advantage of this method is the likelihood that not all prospective patients would be fully insured, or would seek health services. Consequently, it is assumed that where a reduction in the number of patients occurs, the remaining patients would enjoy a proportionate increase in the current facilities. In effect less people would use the same level of facilities.

b. *Wholly Public and Compulsory*

National compulsory insurance is similar to the concept of the national health insurance contributions. A specific contribution from individuals could be used to finance the NHS, and is in effect an earmarked or hypothocated tax. This method of finance would tend to differ only in degree from the existing method. While the details of a such a proposal would require careful thought before introduction, a possible scheme could be that everyone would pay a national health insurance premium, which would be paid directly into the NHS coffers. People in employment could have such premiums deducted from their pay, not only in respect of themselves, but also for their families. Those people not in employment, but dependent on the state, such as pensioners and the unemployed, could contribute by an equivalent contribution from the relevant arm of Government budgets, thus transferring the cost of these citizens to the state. The amount of the premium and any variations for age or sex, would obviously determine the amount to be spent on the NHS and any claim for additional resources would be met from an appropriate increase in the premiums. In such a scheme the corresponding level of health services would still be dependent on political influences. Such a national scheme implies national standard premiums. These contributions may be irrestistible to the tinkerings of Cabinet Ministers and so the NHS would still not be in control of its own financial destiny. Any major advantage over the present method would be lost.

The philosophy of a national compulsory insurance scheme is complementary to a publicly owned health service. However, this is not necessarily fixed. It would be possible to provide a private or mixed health service with this method of finance. However, any private element would almost certainly wish to exert some control over the amount of income it would receive in order to ensure that its costs were at least covered. Such influence may not be acceptable to Governments.

c. *Mix of These Two*

The Royal Commission on the NHS examined this type of mixed insurance scheme as an alternative to the present method and regarded two of the main features as being insurance cover which could be bought from private agencies being combined with an element of choice. The arrangements were seen as being similar to motor insurance, so that a compulsory national minimum level of health insurance would be required, perhaps with premiums varying between clients according to risk, and enhanced policies available by choice. The compulsory minimum could be defined in several ways. For example, it could be a fixed sum for every person or family; or a sum required from people according to their income level, excluding the elderly and chronically sick. The compulsory minimum may exclude cover for personal catastrophe, such as motor accidents, which could be the subject of separate insurance cover. The minimum cover could be arranged from private agencies or from a public government agency. Supplementary cover would tend to be from private agencies.

The main advantage of such a system is often considered to be that more resources would be devoted to health services. However this seems to make huge assumptions about the relationship between price and demand. For example, as premiums rise in real terms, clients may choose to give up the voluntary extra cover and limit premiums to the statutory minimum. Rises in this base premium may be limited by political influence, thus limiting the amount of additional income that can be generated. The precise effect of such reactions cannot be estimated easily due to the lack of information on consumer behaviour in such a hypothetical and as yet unknown market.

The broad approach was revealed as the basis of study by the Government's working party on health service finance. A method similar to that used in some EEC countries such as Germany and Holland was apparently seen as having some potential. Two of the insurance schemes considered were, firstly, a national scheme with a facility to opt out for private cover, and secondly, a scheme which requires employers or trade unions to contribute to part of the cost of health services.

One advantage of such a system is its element of choice. Those paying the higher premiums would perhaps receive better and earlier treatment. Those paying the lower premiums would receive the minimum treatment which may still have to be rationed by some sort of queue, or waiting list, probably longer than at present. Having exercised choice before the onset of illness, patients could not legitimately complain about relative standards of care while receiving treatment. However, such a feature has little to do with determining the acceptable minimum level of care which would be provided to those paying lower premiums. This would be a matter of public policy, not related to the level of premiums.

While this choice may operate adequately for routine medical care, the proposition is quite different for emergency care and the long stay services. In the mixed system many routine cases would probably be dealt with by the private sector, leaving the public sector to finance the emergency and long stay services. Those who claim that compassion would ensure equity may be overlooking the present arrangements where the private sector provision seems to place more emphasis on the lucrative medical treatment rather than on providing a balanced service by including those activities with poor financial returns. Consequently, an imbalanced two-tier service may develop with mixed insurance schemes.

Cost-consciousness on the patient's behalf is also put forward as a justification for insurance based finance. Because patients could pay their health service bills then claim reimbursement, they will eventually know the cost of their treatment. This is seen as a constraint on demands. The incentive to moderate unreasonable demand may be a pious hope when patients have already paid in advance and the cost of their treatment is spread over a large range of premiums. In this respect, insurance based finance does not differ significantly from the present method.

The Royal Commission put forward two disadvantages. First: that some groups in the community would be bad health risks and too poor to pay. These include the elderly, children and the mentally and physically handicapped. An estimated 60% of NHS expenditure is consumed by these types of patient. Second; the cost of administration would be higher than the present system.

This difference can be gauged by comparing the NHS management costs of about 4% with those in EEC countries of between 5% and 10%. On balance, the Royal Commission did not consider that the NHS should be financed by health insurance: a view which we share.

9.5   Partial Charges

Turning from insurance, to the charges to which it relates, brings us into an area which is both varied and controversial. Charges can either be used as a means of financing the NHS or alternatively, they may be used to supplement the resources available to it. It is in this latter respect to which we now turn, so dealing with the second criticism of NHS finance mentioned earlier, that it is due for renovation.

Limited charges for health services have been considered almost since its inception. The 1950 Cabinet papers released by the Public Records Office in January 1981 revealed Aneurin Bevan's opposition to a proposed 50p a week hotel charge which was supported by the Chancellor, Sir Stafford Cripps. Subsequently, in 1951 a compromise was apparently reached and dental and ophthalmic charges were introduced. The debate seems similar to that currently underway in the Government and in the NHS, and as such illustrates the limited scope for supplementary sources of finance and the inevitable lack of imagination that often creeps into the matter. Before considering the extension of charges, a brief outline of the existing charges is appropriate.

Eight main types of charges are levied, three for FPC services and five for hospital services. Charges for FPC services include prescription charges, dental charges and ophthalmic charges.

Hospital charges can be summarised as prescription charges for out-patients together with charges for various wigs and fabric supports; amenity beds for patients requiring private accommodation; private patients charges for accommodation and treatment; income arising from road accidents which is usually paid by insurance companies, and charges for overseas visitors.

These charges have never represented a substantial proportion of NHS resources. However, scope does exist for some increase in income from these sources together with some additional sources but before describing them in detail, we outline some criteria by which these charges may be judged to be accpetable or not. These criteria were recently set down in an article published in the Economist and are as follows: An acceptable charge must:

(a) Maximise the revenue collected;
(b) Minimise administrative costs;
(c) Avoid deterring those patients who, if not treated, will generate extra costs to the NHS in future years;
(d) Try to ensure that charges do not impose the heaviest burden on those who are most seriously ill;
(e) Have exemptions designed so as to avoid accentuating the poverty trap and weakening incentives to work.

The above are a formidable list of criteria and it will clearly be difficult to find a charge that will satisfactorily meet all of the above criteria. Nevertheless we now turn to some specific examples of possible NHS charges:

a. In-Patient Drug Charges

Currently charges are usually made for prescriptions issued by GPs and to hospital out-patients. No charge is made to hospital in-patients. It would seem consistent to extend the prescription charge to such patients, and thus increase the income of the DHAs. Due to the exemption rules, it is difficult to believe that much income could be raised and also administrative costs of collection are likely to be high.

b. Hotel Charges

These have already been briefly mentioned. The argument is that although medical treatment should be provided free, patients should be expected to pay for the costs of maintaining themselves while in hospitals especially as part of the cost would have been paid by the patient himself had he not been in hospital, e.g. food costs. Per patient these hotel costs – catering, laundry, and domestic services – are estimated to be £5 a day at 1981 prices and thus the average patient would pay between £40 - £50 for each stay in hospital. Although such a proposal might generate around £200 million per annum for the NHS, there would be considerable problems in applying it. Although £40 - £50 per stay might not be regarded as unreasonable it would be a large enough sum to cause difficulty to many people. Hence there would be a need for some form of means test with the consequent administrative cost that that would impose. Furthermore there would be difficulty in deciding what to do about long-stay patients such as geriatric patients whose bills could amount to several thousand pounds each year. Such elderly patients occupy some 40% of NHS beds and to exclude them could reduce dramatically the potential income from this source. At the time of writing the Government is against this type of charge.

c. Ambulance Charges

Ambulance services are sometimes used as an alternative to private transport arrangements. In such circumstances it could be argued that the patient could easily make his own arrangements for which he would bear the cost. If the principle was established that patients should contribute to their own transport costs, then income would be generated and almost certainly, costs would be reduced due to lower demand as cheaper alternatives are found. It is difficult to estimate the income that would be raised, but if every journey was charged at a flat rate of say £1, the most that could be collected would be approximately £20 million. However against this would have to be set the costs of income collection.

d. Charges for Overseas Visitors

This is an interesting example as it shows the difficulties of implementing a worthwhile charging method. The levying of charges on overseas visitors has been applied for about two years and what has been observed is that whatever the merits of this approach, the sums involved and the difficulties of collection tend to make it financially unsound for most DHAs. This is especially the case where the number of overseas patients are a very small proportion of the total number of patients, for example in many rural DHAs.

Perhaps such an approach might have been successful had it been applied selectively to certain DHAs where the income collected was likely to be greater than the costs of collection and not applied uniformly across the NHS. The potential income does not seem likely to be anywhere near the original estimate of £6 million a year without significant increases in the unit price.

e. Flat Rate Charge on Hospital/GP Visits

It was recently suggested that the only feasible charging option was to levy a flat rate charge for every visit made to a hospital or a general practitioner and for every day spent in hospital up to a maximum of £50 each year. Exemptions would be given to pregnant women and the under-16s, those being the classes where any deterrent effect of the charge would have damaging long term implications for the nations health. Based on a £2 levy the likely income collected would amount to some £400 million a year. Difficulties of payment could be mitigated by the introduction of NHS stamps which could be purchased in the same way as TV licence stamps.

The authors of the proposal argue that such a charge should not present undue financial hardship on patients and they believe the collection costs of such a system would not exceed a quarter of the additional revenue collected. Based on our experience of financial systems we would be rather sceptical of the latter claim without further detailed examination.

An important consideration in partial charging is its *raison d'etre*. As mentioned earlier, in our opinion, the present Government tends to see it as a means of reducing public spending. An alternative approach urges the introduction of partial charges in order to create more resources for the NHS. Yet another believes it to be desirable because it is a fairer way to finance the NHS while a fourth sees it as important in influencing the behaviour of both patients and staff. Conclusions derived from an appraisal of charging in the NHS will differ depending on the aim of the charges, and it is always important to bear this is mind. Gains in respect of one approach can often represent disadvantages in another, and a careful balance should always be strived for. For example, if it is intended to increase income, those less well off and generally more needy may be unable to find the increased cost and would therefore be unable to seek the benefit of health services. This may be seen as an unacceptable implication.

Management costs are also a major consideration. It is clearly not sound to proceed with a proposal to collect partial charges if the administrative costs will exceed the income collected. This factor must be reflected very carefully both in the type of charge and its amount. For example, some partial charges may not be viable at all, while others may only be viable above a certain level. In this respect, principles have to be balanced with pragmatism.

One major consideration with partial charges, and indeed other charges, is the method of fixing their levels. Two main approaches can be called the central and the local. The central approach would result in nationally applied charges being levied in all DHAs, irrespective of the associated costs. This would result in patients paying the same charges for the same service in all parts of the country. DHAs would have the task of ensuring that a loss would not be made on the services or that the subsidy would not be excessive.

The alternative would be for DHAs to fix their own partial charges. Thus differing local costs would be reflected in differing local charges. The principle of autonomy in fixing charges is not commonly used in the NHS. However, one major advantage is that locally determined charges would reflect the fact that similar services provided by DHAs are never precisely the same. In these circumstances, slightly differing charges could be justified. However, the introduction of such an approach would have to be based on a consistent methodology in the way that the charges are calculated. This local approach would also reflect the viability of charges. For example, if, in a particular DHA, the administrative cost of collecting standard charges from overseas visitors exceeds the income, then the charges could either be waived or be increased to reflect the administrative costs. Flexibility is the attraction of the local approach.

9.6 Supplementary Income

Supplementary sources of income have recently presented themselves to the NHS. The Health Services Act 1980 and subsequently health circular HC(80)11 gives DHAs the opportunity to raise voluntary money to supplement that already raised and donated to the NHS by organisations such as the League of Friends. The specific arrangements are extremely limited and it is important to bear this in mind. DHAs fund raising activities should be self financing, with administrative and similar costs being met from the proceeds. Thus, any initial expenses met from exchequer or trust funds are effecively an interest free loan and have to be repaid from the proceeds as a first charge. Any surplus should then be held in trust for the purpose for which it was given.

The types of fund raising activities permitted are limited to fetes, bazaars and collections. Specifically excluded are lotteries of the type available to local authorities and other gaming activities associated with bingo halls, casinos, and gaming clubs. However, similar small scale activities such as raffles are permitted where they form a small part of the total fund raising event, such as a fete. In addition to these legal restrictions, unsuitable activities are discouraged which may bring the NHS into disrepute, for example, using cigarette and alcohol as raffle prizes. Sponsorship also presents ethical problems. Direct blatant advertising by sponsors should generally be discouraged and the NHS should not appear to be promoting any particular product, especially tobacco, alcohol, or medical products.

The circular also includes provision for co-operation with existing voluntary bodies, and this general arrangement was all that the voluntary bodies expected. When health circular HC(80)11 was issued the Secretary of State was subject to criticism by the voluntary bodies. In particular, they pressed for a similar interest free loan for their initial expenses and the removal of the threat of a NHS takeover.

The potential for local and specific appeals should not be under-estimated. For example, in a number of towns, appeals for funds to purchase body scanners have resulted in sums of the order of £½ million being collected. However, it is important to realise that such monies are only available to meet the initial capital cost of such equipment. The annual costs of operating such equipment are not the subject of such appeals and must be financed by the DHA itself from its own resources. Consequently, it is important for DHAs to influence the efforts of the voluntary bodies, especially when the recurring revenue consequences can be significant and DHAs may become morally committed to them.

One other possible source of income in NHS finance is selling surplus land. The selling of land could produce a useful injection of additional finance resulting in an increase of non-recurring monies. The sums to be realised would depend on each DHA completing a comprehensive review of the land in its district, together with an appropriately devised policy by each RHA which allowed DHAs to retain the benefit of such arrangements. A recent report (the Ceri Davies Report) has addressed the issue of under-utilised holdings of land and buildings by DHAs. Several recommendations were made emphasising that health authorities should pay more attention to the value of their estate.

To conclude this chapter, we wish to remind readers that changing the method of finance of health services is not synonymous with an increase in the resources available, nor does it automatically infer improved levels of service with more patients being treated. Similarly, transferring part or all of the cost of the NHS from the public purse to the paying patient does not necessarily mean that the taxpayer would receive a full refund. Such matters would be settled by Government policy and the commercial climate of any element of private health service.

10

Improving Efficiency in the National Health Service

10.1 Introduction

In Chapter 9, we briefly mentioned that one way to ease the pressure on NHS resources was to use those resources in a more efficient manner. Clearly efficiency is very topical in all parts of the public sector, including the NHS, and in this chapter we wish to pursue it in a little more depth. Thus our aim will be to discuss four issues:

(a) what precisely is meant by efficiency;
(b) how greater efficiency may be pursued;
(c) the scope for improved efficiency in the NHS;
(d) the effect of greater decentralised internal financing.

In discussing the scope for improving efficiency in the NHS, we will draw on examples to illustrate the point but those examples must not be thought of as an exhaustive list.

10.2 The Meaning of Efficiency

We believe the term efficiency is too loosely banded about in the public sector these days. A variety of people use the term while attaching different meanings to it and frequently confusing effectiveness with efficiency. Therefore it will first be useful to clarify the meaning of the two terms for the purpose of our analysis:

a. Effectiveness

This is concerned with the progress made by a person or organisation towards some pre-determined objective. It is really a measure of how successfully or otherwise particular activities are actually being performed. Thus it is not directly concerned with the resources being put into that activity. An NHS example could be the effectiveness of different forms of clinical practice. Let us assume that our aim is to reduce peri-natal mortality by some pre-determined amount. If it could be shown that one form of clinical practice achieved this aim to a greater degree than another form, then we would say the former was more effective than the latter, irrespective of the costs involved in each case. Similarly advances in medical technology can make a service more effective even though it can increase the costs. The problem with measuring effectiveness is that it is linked to the measurement of the 'output' of health services. The difficulties of measuring output are discussed in Chapter 7.

b. Efficiency

If effectiveness is concerned with how well an activity is performed, efficiency is concerned with how cheaply it is done. However the cheapest activity is not necessarily the most efficient as we have also to take account of both the quantity and quality of the output of the activity. In a formal manner, we could describe efficiency as shown below:

$$\text{Efficiency of activity} = \frac{\text{Costs incurred on activity}}{\text{Units of output obtained}}$$

Thus we cannot measure efficiency unless we capture information about costs and are able to measure output. We cannot state that one activity is more efficient than another unless we can also measure what those activities actually produce in output terms. However, in practice, we have to be a little more realistic and make some broad assumptions about the output of activities if we are to make any headway in the search for efficiency. For example, we assume that the unit costs of food is an indicator of catering efficiency even though it is possible to argue that this takes no account of the standard of the meals produced. However, the point about output should not be overlooked when considering efficiency measures.

What has been said above leads us on to the next point about the link between true efficiency and reductions in the cost of providing activities. Too often it is blandly assumed that if expenditure on public services is reduced, this automatically implies that greater efficiency has been achieved. The discussion above should convince the reader that such expenditure savings can just as easily come about as a result of cuts in the effectiveness of those services as from greater efficiency. This leads us on to a general rule-of-thumb to be used when assessing or searching for greater efficiency. Greater efficiency can be said to have been achieved where:

(a) the same amount and standards of services are produced for less cost;
(b) improved amounts and/or standards of services are produced for the same cost;
(c) a more useful activity is substituted for a less useful one at the same cost;
(d) needless activities are eliminated.

Although it still begs the question as to how standard of service should be measured, the above statements should always be borne in mind when discussing the topic of efficiency.

10.3   The Search for Efficiency

It is a commonly held assumption that if we need to produce greater efficiency in the NHS, all we have to do is cut the resources available and greater efficiency will be the result. As we have already argued, the result of such an approach is just as likely to be a cut in services. It cannot be emphasised too strongly that improvements in efficiency can only be obtained by searching for it and such a search requires considerable managerial effort. Nor should the topic of efficiency be regarded as something transitory. The search for greater efficiency should be regarded as the apothesis of good management and should be pursued at all times and not just as a response to exhortation of the government of the day.

10.4   Systems Versus In-Depth Reviews

In considering how the quest for improved efficiency should be pursued, we would suggest that there are two possible approaches, namely the use of systems and the use of in-depth reviews. However, it is important to note that the distinction between these two approaches is not always clear cut.

a. Systems

In an organisation such as a DHA there will be a variety of systems in operation to facilitate the management of the organisation. Some of these systems might be complex and orientated around a computer while others may be simple and manual in operation. Examples of such systems might be purchasing systems, investment appraisal systems, and budgeting systems. Some of these systems, and their potential contribution to improved efficiency, have been discussed in earlier chapters.

Perhaps the most topical system of all would be manpower information systems since there has been considerable and probably merited criticism of

NHS manpower control. One way of promoting efficiency would be to review the adequacy and use made of all these systems and to implement improvements where necessary. If such systems are found to be adequate in nature and are being properly used by managers, then it is reasonable to assume that optimal efficiency is being obtained. However, if this is not the case then improvements in the design and use of systems should lead to improved efficiency. We delay until later the question of who should carry out such system reviews.

b. In-Depth Reviews

The alternative approach would be to choose a particular activity in the DHA and to conduct an in-depth review of that activity with the aim of improving efficiency. Such a review would aim to answer the following questions:

(i) Why is the activity done at all?
(ii) Why is it done the way it is?
(iii) Could it be done in an alternative manner?
(iv) Which of the alternatives outlined is the best one?

The surgical services of a DHA with its complex relationships between out-patients, day patients, theatre, and in-patient services, together with the range of support services, provide an excellent example of a topic for a regular in-depth review. Changes in medical technology, surgical techniques, and nursing practices, mean that some of the existing services could become obsolete while others could become overloaded and suffer from bottlenecks in throughput. Asking each of the four questions above in a constructive manner could well produce greater efficiency as we have defined it.

Clearly there is a limit to how many in-depth reviews can be carried out by a DHA in any one year and thus much of effort of improving efficiency should rest on the systems review. However both approaches are valid and should be used in an appropriate manner.

10.5   Requirements of an Efficiency Search

If a search for improved efficiency is to be carried out, we suggest that there are two necessary pre-requisites:

(a) Sufficient managerial input
(b) Adequate information.

We shall consider each these in turn.

10.6 Sufficient Managerial Input

We have already made the point that gains in efficiency will not be achieved without effort on behalf of management. We believe that the whole thrust of the Griffiths Inquiry was on the need to improve the general management process at both district and unit level and hence to obtain increased efficiency. However this managerial input does not have to come directly from the health authorities own management but could derive from external sources. We discuss below some ways in which the search for improved efficiency could be conducted.

b. External Consultants

The DHA could engage a firm of management consultants or an organis-ation like the Management Advisory Service of the NHS. In most consult-ancy firms the consultants employed would be of a high calibre and would have experience drawn from many different organisations. Thus they would have an awareness of what constitutes current good practice. However, it is usually thought desirable that the consultancy firm employed should have an awareness of the environment and complexities of the NHS and many firms are now able to offer the services of health service specialists. The main disadvantage in using management consult-ants is that they can be costly and thus the DHA might be involved in considerable expense.

We would anticipate that management consultants would be likely to emphasise systems, throughput and organisational aspects of efficiency.

b. Inter-Authority Reviews

The suggestion has been made that DHAs might improve their efficiency by the use of inter-authority reviews. The idea is that the managers of one DHA might review the activities of a neighbouring DHA, the hope being that a fresh set of minds might more easily identify efficiency improve-ments.

Whatever the merits of this idea, it seems unlikely that many managers will have sufficient time left over from managing their own DHA to devote to reviews of another. Furthermore, this approach would have to be handled with great sensitivity.

c. Matrix Group

The matrix group is a particular form of organisation that can usefully be applied to the search for greater efficiency. The matrix group comprises a group of individuals from several disciplines who meet periodically to study a particular matter in depth. Most of their working week will be spent working within their own department but for say a half a day per week the individuals might come together as a group to search for improved efficiency in a particular area. Thus the group will have the benefit of multi-disciplinary expertise.

We believe the matrix group method has been utilised in the NHS for many years though perhaps not always with the aim of pursuing greater efficiency. The existence of unit management in health authorities should be conducive to this approach.

d. *VFM teams*

There have been many suggestions for the creation of such VFM teams, at RHA or DHA level, who would pursue the search for greater efficiency. Such teams might or might not be part of an internal audit department.

We are a little sceptical of this development. By definition such VFM teams would not have a detailed knowledge of the workings of an individual department nor would they have the range of experience of the external consultant. Thus we do not believe such teams could come up with much more then very general recommendations.

In summary, we would wish to see the thrust of efficiency studies to take place at unit level, possibly by the use of matrix groups. Initially there would also seem to be scope for the use of outside expertise especially in the systems area.

10.7   Adequate Information

However such an efficiency search might be conducted, it is likely that it will be hamstrung by the absence of adequate information on which to conduct any investigation. The NHS is frequently criticised for the poor range and quality of the information it produces but we believe this is due, at least in part, to the lack of investment in up-to-date information systems. The Korner recommendations on information have clearly given a boost to the topic of information production in the NHS. However, it remains to be seen whether the large investment in the information systems necessitated by the Korner proposals will be forthcoming.

10.8   Potential Scope for Improving Efficiency

In this section it is not our intention to try and give an exhaustive catalogue of potential efficiency savings in the NHS. Rather we just wish to touch on a few areas where there would appear to be considerable scope for improving efficiency given the definition of efficiency outlined in 10.2. The topics are only briefly discussed and the interested reader is referred to the references for further details.

a. Purchasing Arrangements

The NHS as a whole spends huge amounts on a variety of supplies and it is clear that even small economies of say 1%, in this area, could produce large cash savings. Furthermore the sheer size of the NHS means that it should have immense bargaining power to ensure good prices are obtained for products pruchased. The creation of the NHS Supplies Council has clearly resulted in a greater importance being given to the area of NHS purchasing. Since its inception the NHS Supplies Council has been very active in assessing the adequacy of the purchasing function in RHAs and in improving national purchasing on behalf of the NHS as a whole, especially with the introduction of the Supplies Information System.

The problem in deciding the best purchasing arrangements for a health authority is that there will always be a trade-off between the following positions:

(i)   Greater centralisation of purchasing should lead to lower prices being obtained but will also require greater standardisation of items purchaded with a consequent reduction in the lines purchased.

(ii) Less centralisation of purchasing will probably mean higher prices being paid but will require less standardisation of the items purchased and hence more likelihood that the items purchased will meet the needs of the user.

In the case of items such as fuel where there can be little variation in product specification, there is clearly a case for national purchasing and this is indeed what happens. In the case of other items it is important not to be dogmatic. It is for the health authorities themselves to work out the best purchasing arrangements for each item be it at regional, district or sub district level. A balance must be struck between price of the product and the suitability of that product. A word of caution must be that DHAs should not reject a more centralised purchasing arrangement for certain items just because the greater standardisation of those items does not fit in with the idiosyncrasies of certain professions within the NHS.

Finally we would wish to emphasise the distinction between centralised purchasing and centralised storage of supplies. Each is important and has its own conribution to make to improved efficiency but they should not be confused and each should be judged separately on its own merits.

b. Tendering for Support Services

We believe that this is an issue which, in recent years, has been portrayed as a great ideological conflict and as such has generated great heat and little light. The central issue is clear cut: *is it an acceptable managerial option to invite tenders for the provision of certain support services such as catering and cleaning from external contractors?* The answer to this question must clearly be yes when it can be shown that the advantages of doing so outweigh the disadvantages. The difficulty with tendering is not one of principle but one of managerial judgement about the merits of the options available.

Health authorities are requested to periodically obtain tenders for the provision of support services. Such tenders would be sought from external companies and from the in-house organisation. Again we see nothing wrong in principle with health authorities widening their options by testing the market for the provision of such services. Indeed we would emphasise that where external provision of support services currently takes place, the health authority should periodically review the situation to see if contracting-in to a direct labour department might be a better option. However, before any decision is taken a rigorous appraisal of the various options must be undertaken and, in our opinion, it is in this appraisal process that the circular is weak. It is simplistic to suppose that decision between internal and external provision of support services can be made purely on the basis of lowest tender price.

When analysing various options for the provision of support services the following should be taken into account:-

(i)   *Costs* – the costs of each option in both the short and long term should be taken into account. Furthermore an attempt must be made to identify any hidden costs. As an example here we have the need for DHAs to employ additional staff to monitor volumes and standards of services when contracting out a laundry service.

(ii) *Effects of Inflation* – the major factor influencing future costs of in-house services would be the national wage agreement for staff. The health authority cash limits provide, at least in part, for such increases. Consideration would need to be given to the impact of inflation if such services were provided by an external contractor. For example, *would* the contractor be prepared to restrict any price increases to that allowed for the inflation in cash limits?

(iii) *Quality of Service* – *what would be the impact on the quality of service provided by each option?* This is a very complex question and we would need to look at a whole variety of factors which can be regarded as contributing to quality of service. For example, the following are important:

- Period of service – *over what period is the service provided? Is it just provided during the working day or is there a night service or a weekend service?*
- Standard of service – *to what standard is the service to be provided?*
- Flexibility of service – *how flexible will the service provision be? Will it be tightly scheduled or will it be on demand?*

(iv) *Control of Standards* – what does the management of the health authority have over the standards of service provision? With an in-house service they clearly have direct managerial control but with external provision the position is not so clear cut. Although a contract would exist between the health authority and the contractor it is not always easy to enforce such a contract. In extreme cases the health authority might find itself involved in extensive litigation in trying to prove that the terms of the contract have not been complied with. While such an argument is continuing, one might rightly question what is happening to the service standards.

(v) *Longer Term Implications* – the health authority should consider the likely longer term implications of contracting out support services. If the external contractor selected proves unsatisfactory it is essential that the authority has other options available for the longer term.
Two questions arise directly from this:
- *Would it be feasible for the authority to once more contract-in the service?* This may not always be feasible especially where a large capital investment would be required.
- *Would alternative contractors be available and capable of taking on the service possibly at very short notice?*

c. Impact of New Technology

Health authorities in common with most public services are labour intensive with labour costs amounting to some 75% of total expenditure. As a general point we would imagine that there must be considerable scope in the NHS for the use of the new micro-technology as a substitute for labour. More specifically we see this as being applicable in the administrative field. For a number of years there has been criticism of the size of administrative costs in the NHS. Although we believe these criticisms to be largely unfounded there would seem to be scope for automating many administrative procedures thereby reducing administrative costs still further. As some examples of ways in which this might be done we quote the following:

(i)   word processors
(ii) electronic mail
(iii) information storage and retrieval – especially in the field of medical records
(iv) information manipulation.

There are clealry a number of formidable barriers to the introduction of the above. There would be considerable opposition from trade unions and the medical profession. However, this does not mean an attempt should not be made and indeed there are several pilot studies already being carried out in the NHS.

10.9   The Effect of Greater Decentralised Internal Financing

The Griffiths Inquiry's main thrust is seen as improving the general management of the NHS and it is important to recognise that any changes will be limited without a revision of the NHS internal financing arrangements. In particular, greater de-centralisation of financing, which would require DHAs to pay for the consequences of more of their managerial actions would be beneficial. Three main areas of change would be in the areas of bank balances, stock holdings and capital finance. These are considered below.

a. Bank Balances

Currently the cost of holding high bank balances, low creditor balances and high debtor balances is financed centrally by the Treasury. It is easy to identify the lack of incentive to DHAs to be efficient in the management of such balances as inefficiency carries no cost penalty.

It would be relatively easy to introduce an arrangement which would be internal to the NHS by which DHAs had to bear the cost of inefficient levels of balances by requiring them to finance their arrangements. This would be most easily achieved by changing the banking arrangements so that DHAs could manage their funds by seeking interest on high bank balances and having to finance overdrafts. This commercial approach would bring with it the advantages of commercial management and is therefore consistent with the Government's aim.

One difficulty with the approach is that in the interests of national efficiency, DHAs would have to be prevented from drawing excessive volumes of cash from the DHSS and placing these on deposit in order to increase the resources available to it. This could be achieved by fixing a maximum bank balance for each DHA any over-shoot would result in financial penalties.

Alternatively, the DHSS could charge DHAs for the cash drawn each day. This cost could then be recovered by the DHA by prudent commercial management of its bank balance.

b. Stockholdings

As for bank balances, DHAs carry no penalty for carrying high or inappropriate stocks nor do they receive any benefit by managing these efficiently. If the internal financing arrangements were changed by introducing a more commercial approach which required DHAs to finance their stockholding costs it is clear that DHAs would be motivated to manage their stocks more efficiently to order to optimise their financial implications.

Such an approach should also strengthen the role of the Supplies Council which has made significant strides in improving the daily management of supplies. It would also be consistent with the Management Inquiry's objectives.

c. Capital Finance

To a DHA capital is a free good. DHAs pay no interest and capital finance can be seen as a grant from the DHSS. It would be consistent with the moves towards better investment appraisal and better general management if DHAs were to bear the cost of capital as would a commercial undertaking.

One way forward would be to give DHAs their capital cash limits which would be available as loans. As they require capital to finance projects then loans could be made to each DHA by the RHA or DHSS. The interest and principle repayments could be recycled in order to increase DHAs revenue cash limits to provide additional revenue finance for the capital repayments. This approach is similar in part to that envisaged by the bidding approach described in the RAWP report.

The major advantage of this decentralised capital financing is that DHAs would have to bear the full cost of both revenue and capital developments. It would then be able to take these into account in determining priorities. With the present method, capital solutions to problems can often be given undue preference because of the cheapness of capital.

d. Objectives

The usual objectives to such changes are that they are not in the interests of national objectives to managing public expenditure. Our response to this criticism would be that until such a decentralised approach is tried the actual effect at the national level cannot be fully assessed. Furthermore, *would the aggregate national improvements in general management outweigh the disadvantages of perhaps more difficult national financial control?* To test the effect an experiment perhaps in two regions may provide evidence of the relative benefits. Our view is that if it is appropriate to operate financial management at the budgetholder or clinician level in the NHS it is appropriate to move the internal financing arrangements from the national level to the more local level of the DHA.

One other criticism of the decentralised approach is the view that Treasurers should be operating efficient levels of balances and financing anyway because it represents good practice. Our response to that approach is that DHAs should be providing good general management because it is good practice but by implication the establishment of the Griffiths Inquiry indicate that the Government are not satisfied with the assumption. *Why should it be satisfied with assumptions about internal financing arrangements?*

Bibliography

This brief bibliography is intended as a guide for the interested reader who wishes to delve further into various aspects of NHS management and finance. The list should be regarded as illustrative and not exhaustive.

General Works
(1) Report of the Royal Commission on the NHS Cmnd 7615, (HMSO)
(2) Research paper No 2 of the Royal Commission on the NHS 'Management of Financial Resources in the NHS' (HMSO 1978)
(3) 'Crisis in the Health Service the Politics of Management' Alasgeweki A. and Haywood S. (Croon Helm 1980)
(4) 'Priorities for Health and Social Services' Bevan G., et al. (Croon Helm 1980)
(5) 'Hospital Beds: A Problem for Diagnosis and Management' Yates J. (Heinemann 1982)
(6) Financial Information Service (Volume 30-Health) (Chartered Institute of Public Finance and Accountancy)
(7) Health Care UK 1984 – An Economic Social and Policy Audit (Chartered Institute of Public Finance and Accountancy 1984)

Resource Allocation
(1) Research Paper No. 3 of the Royal Commission on the NHS 'Allocating Health Resource; A Commentary on the Report of the Resource Allocation Working Party' (HMSO 1978)
(2) 'Sharing Resources for Health in England; Report of the Resource Allocation Working Party' DHSS (HMSO 1976)
(3) 'Report of the Advisory Group on Resource Allocation' DHSS (AGRA 1980)
(4) From Principles to Practice; A Commentary on Health Service Planning and Resource Allocation in England from 1970 to 1980' Butts M., et al. (Nuffield Provisional Hospitals Trust 1981)

Planning
(1) 'Policy Making and Planning in the Health Sector' Lee K. and Mills A. (Croon Helm 1981)
(2) Op cit, Butts M. et al.

206

Financial Control
(1) 'Public Sector Accounting and Financial Control' Henley D., et al. (Van Nostrand Reinhold 1983)
(2) 'Public Sector Accounting' Jones R. and Pendlebury M. (Pitmans 1984)
(3) Health Service Value for Money Guide Chartered Institute of Public Finance and Accountancy 1984)

Index